The Reflex Relaxation Response

– JAMES BROCKBANK –

An environmentally friendly book printed and bound in England by www.printondemand-worldwide.com

FSC Mixed Sources
Product group from well-managed forests, and other controlled sources
www.fsc.org Cert no. TT-COC-002641
© 1996 Forest Stewardship Council

PEFC Certified
This product is from sustainably managed forests and controlled sources
www.pefc.org
PEFC/16-33-415

This book is made entirely of chain-of-custody materials

FastPrint Publishing

www.fast-print.net/store.php

The reflex Relaxation Response

ISBN 978-178035-071-4

First published 2011 by
FASTPRINT PUBLISHING
Peterborough, England.

Also by James Brockbank

One Without Shame

Head to Foot

Post-Traumatic Stress

Something Special

Badger Killer

Reflex-Relaxology

Dedicated to Reflexologists

Whilst the advice and information in this book are believed to be accurate neither the author nor the publisher can accept any legal responsibility for any injury sustained whilst following any of the suggestions made herein.

Contents

Introduction

My interest in reflexology began in 1959. I was a young National Service soldier on active service abroad. This involved a great deal of what we termed "foot slogging" over some very rough mountainous terrain. My feet were not accustomed to so much hard walking and became sore and painful. So breaks during "foot slogging" patrols were used to take of my boots and massage the feet. I found this exercise remarkable, not only because it eased my painful feet, but also gave me some relief from a sinus problem.

Some years later, during my student days, I read a book called "Stories the Feet can Tell" written by Eunice Ingham. As a result, a lifelong interest and research into reflexology began. Doreen Bayly, a student of Eunice Ingham's, introduced reflexology to Great Britain in the early sixties, although it was not until the eighties that it became well known in this country.

At this time I was the headmaster of a special school and able to observe physiotherapists occasionally using reflexology. They combined it as part of their work with children in the special care unit attached to the school. This reinforced my fascination in the therapy. In particular I was convinced of its use for treating stress.

After retiring I found my interest could not be appeased without qualifying as a practitioner. I then became a lecturer in its possibilities for relieving stress.

During this time, I became convinced that certain reflex points should be studied and recorded for their relaxing benefits. These are the reflexes, which make up, "Reflex-Relaxology".

This book covers the practicalities of a study for which I have to thank my mentor and advisor Dr. Joseph Friend, also recipients using the treatment. They gave me the encouragement and inspiration to write the book.

The writing isn't meant to be a textbook of reflexology. It attempts to demonstrate a simple technique that can be learned by a whole family. It is a very safe method, but as with any form of complementary therapy, consult your doctor before deciding if it is appropriate for any condition you may have and be aware of any contraindications.

Chapter One

Reflex-Relaxology (R.R.)

Relaxation is at your feet

Reflex-Relaxology (referred to as R.R. throughout the book) is based on the principles of reflexology. It uses the same reflexes as traditional reflexology and follows its basic philosophy. However, R.R. therapy is a total concentration on achieving relaxation by calming the nervous system and linking psychological with physical benefits. It consists of using the hands to work on sixteen reflex points on the soles of the feet. The fingers or thumbs give a gentle pressure to the specific points with the aim of creating a soothing effect, and at the same time improving blood flow to the whole body.

As a therapist you can perfect a sensitive awareness of touch and a capacity to heal, and as a receiver you are able to gain a more responsive ability for healing to take place.

Before giving treatment it is important to receive instruction and guidance from a professional reflexologist. If you do not understand what you are doing you could overwork a reflex area that results in disturbing the balance in the body.

Once you become competent in the knowledge and practice of the therapy, view it as, not merely a self-help exercise, but as a skill that can benefit your family and friends. It is a means by which you can, if you wish, foster richer family and social relationships.

Through practice, a gradual sensitivity is built up and you become increasingly aware of what the method can achieve in restoring harmony through relaxation therapy.

Recipient Not Patient

A further explanation is perhaps needed as to why I use the term recipient, (defined in the dictionary as beneficiary or receiver). I do so because as a practitioner I do not refer to those receiving treatment as patients. The word implies someone is ill. A stressed out person is not necessarily ill, although his or her stress may lead to illness. There are many reasons why a person feels the therapy helps them, and for this reason, both in my treatments and lectures I prefer to call those having treatment as recipients.

Development of reflexology

There is not a great deal of knowledge regarding the history of reflexology. Although artefacts and ancient manuscripts give explicit details of pressure points on the feet being treated to heal the body. There is also evidence that the therapy was used, alongside acupuncture, by the Chinese 5000 years ago. Further reference to reflexology techniques can be found on many drawings left by the ancient Egyptians in 3000 BC.

Real documentation did not appear until 1582 with the publication of a book by the physicians Dr Adamus and Dr A'tatis, and a book published in Leipzig by a Dr Bell. Much of these authors' ideas would probably have come from ancient sources.

The concept of reflexology, as we know it today came into prominence in 1917 with the publication of a book called Zone Therapy, or Relieving pain at Home. A Dr. William Fitzgerald who consequently is reputed to have introduced reflexology to western society in the 1900's wrote it. He had been working at the Central London Ears, Nose and Throat Hospital as a consultant before moving to America. His experiments consisted of using pressure on areas of the body to give the patient an anaesthetic effect in a corresponding part of the body. For guidelines he divided the body into ten vertical zones, five on each side of the body. The ten zones were seen as "energy channels" ending in the hands and feet. Dr. Fitzgerald observed pain in a specific part of the body could be alleviated by applying pressure in another part of the body, within the same zone. He believed that it was possible to work on reflexes throughout the body. Most reflexologists concentrate on the feet only although it can be used on the hands. Dr Fitzgerald also believed in health education and emphasised the importance of diet and exercise to reinforce the healing power of zone therapy.

The whole process was developed in much more detail by Eunice Ingham who is credited with "mapping" out the whole body on the feet. The growth of reflexology in the West is due to her. She did research studies as a pupil of Dr Joe Riley, a promoter of Dr Fitzgerald's work. In 1938 she wrote the book 'Stories the Feet can Tell'. Her main perceptions were that the foot "mirrored" tension in a related part of the body and by treating the whole foot there was a relaxing and healing effect on the entire body.

A student of Eunice Ingham, Doreen Bayly was mainly responsible for introducing reflexology into Britain in the early 1960's. She began the now well-established Bayly School of Reflexology.

Chapter Two

How does it work?

There is, as yet, no scientific evidence available that gives a definitive reason as to why reflexology works. Some of the theories put forward are as follows; we no longer walk barefoot so the feet do not receive massage from stones underfoot which normally would have boosted the circulation and massaged away the waste debris from the body which accumulates in the feet.

Dr. Fitzgerald believed that problems in the feet meant the body's organs were not working correctly. So if the area on the foot corresponding to the organ area on the body was massaged correct functioning could take place. He believed that by using a specific type of massage on particular areas of the foot it released an electric nerve impulse that could stimulate the part of the body needing treatment. Looking at this scientifically there is no anatomical link between the foot's reflexes and the internal organs.

A further theory is that reflexology is similar to acupuncture although the principles are different. To some extent reflexology is thought, like acupuncture, to open up blocked energy pathways. This is the oriental idea of energy currents complementing each other, or yin and yang. Kirlian photography (which is reported to show proof of energy fields in the body) has been used to show distinct improvement in the body's energy fields after reflexology.

A popular theory among practitioners is they can treat the lymphatic system by removing toxins from the body. Lymph is a fluid, watery in appearance, contained in the tissues and organs of the body. It is a possibility that reflexology may help to clear toxins and strengthen the immune system.

There is some evidence to suggest that it can release blockages in the nerve endings. This might be caused by uric acid build up in the feet preventing proper circulation of blood and lymph. Therefore, when the deposits are removed circulation is healthier.

How reflexology works cannot rule out the placebo effect which is the psychological theory that it is all in the mind. Meaning a person's illness improves when they believe healing and well-being is taking place.

Of all the many theories put forward, I favour without doubt, the 'relaxation effect' and throughout this book concentrate on what I term reflex- relaxology.

Numerous studies have proven that reflexology is calming and relaxing which helps the body become more effective in counteracting illness.

Through many years of practising and studying reflexology I have found a relaxation response can be gained mainly from the sixteen reflex points making up reflex-relaxology. The points of course link up to the full reflexology map and I am not suggesting that the full treatment is redundant.

Questions commonly asked.

What are the practitioner's qualifications?

He/she should have studied at one of the accredited schools, such as the Bayly School. During their training they should have achieved a sound knowledge of anatomy and physiology, and be skilled in using the practical technique.

At the end of their training, they should pass both theory and practical exams. An unqualified reflexologist cannot gain insurance cover. So check to see if he/she is insured.

What happens in a reflexology session?

The reflexologist begins by making the recipient comfortable, usually in a reclining chair, with their shoes and socks off. He/she will begin the treatment by asking questions about their past medical history which he will carefully note. The treatment is based on a holistic approach to looking at illness and an assessment of one's whole life-style is made during the first visit.

Before beginning the actual therapy, the feet should be examined for callous's, cuts, and other impediments that might mean chiropody would be more appropriate. Depending upon this initial analysis the reflexologist proceeds to use a systematic method of working all the reflex areas on both feet. The whole process takes about one hour

What kind of illness can reflexology help?

A professional reflexologist will not pretend that it is a cure-all on its own. It is used mainly as a supplement along with other treatments. This makes it a matter for conjecture regarding any improvement in a illness. Was it due to reflexology or other therapy? However in the hands of a well trained practitioner with a knowledge of anatomy and physiology it can give relief from many conditions such as back pain, migraine, asthma, sinus pain, depression and stress related problems. Most illness will benefit from a course of reflexology.

Is the treatment painful?

If the treatment is painful, change your therapist. A reflexologist should have sensitive trained hands that are able to apply gentle pressure to the feet and find very tiny deposits that may block energy pathways, if not removed. Neglected areas on the feet can be painful to the touch because they affect muscles and nerves. There are many factors involved in the relationship between the feet and the rest of the body. Any type of foot problem can be detrimental to good health.

What are crystal deposits?

They are thought to be calcium deposits. Possibly caused by excess acidity in the bloodstream. Although this theory has never really been proved. Reflexologists make it an important part of their work to break down the deposits in order to prevent a restriction of normal blood circulation.

It is possible that the tension caused by stress as some effect in contributing to the accumulation of the deposits. A further factor is that the feet are at the bottom of the body's circulatory and waste removal systems.

If I am taking medication, can I have Reflexology?

If you have any illness, before having treatment from a reflexologist, or any therapist, you should take advice from your Doctor. He or she might be able to refer you to one working in their clinic. Do not be afraid to ask for proof of the therapists training, and which registering body, they belong to. Complementary therapies have their own official registering bodies.

Above all, do not terminate any conventional medication you may be taking.

What will the Reflexologist want to know about me?

On your first visit to a practitioner he/she will want to note down any past and present medical conditions or illness. This must be done before a decision can be made as to the suitability of the treatment for your particular case.

Because the therapy is holistic do not be surprised at questions being asked about your life-style.

What is the relevance of the Metamorphic Technique to reflexology?

The metamorphic technique is attributed to a reflexologist called Robert St John who practised the technique in the 1960s, although the way it is practised now and the results aimed for are very much different to reflexology today.

The system works in the belief that many illnesses can be traced back to the prenatal period and these prenatal stages correspond to areas on the foot. A metamorphic practitioner presses the areas to help the healing process. They also work on the head and hands of a recipient.

The technique strongly advocates the holistic approach to the treatment of the body as a whole and not as separate parts. It emphasises a belief that everyone as the potential to heal themselves. The practitioner of the metamorphic technique takes the view that he or she is working as a catalyst and the recipient's life force will do what is correct for their well-being.

During my work in special education, I encountered parents who had taken their handicapped children for treatment by metamorphic practitioners. It is supposed to be useful in treating children with Down's syndrome, brain damage and types of developmental disorders.

Is Reflex-Relaxology different to Reflexology?

It uses the principles of reflexology to educate a person into awareness for healing on two levels, the physiological and psychological. Science has proven that tension is the underlying cause in many physical and mental diseases. It can have devastating effects on the general health and the functioning of the body.

For example, in my experience of schoolchildren's problems I have no doubt that failure to release tension has resulted in delinquency. R.R. helps the individual free mind and body from tension. More than this, it can help the whole family to assist each other in a commitment to achieving a better quality of life.

The concept of the idea should be seen as a skill to gain relaxation, for either oneself or other recipients. It is formulated to give a method of working reflexes on the feet or hands which will relax the body and invigorate the circulation.

What is the main benefit from reflex-relaxology?

By using a simple technique, it brings relaxation to the body and mind. The method is concerned with individuals doing something practical to help themselves.

No apparatus is needed and it can be undertaken in the home. It becomes a tool to counteract stress.

Is the therapy good for anything other than stress?

Stress is responsible for many body reactions, which include high blood pressure, indigestion, stomach disorders and ulcers. So if you are able to gain relaxation from using R.R. you could, to a certain extent, be giving yourself some preventive health care.

Do I need to work on both feet when using R.R.?

Yes, you must remember that one foot represents half the body. And although in R.R. you are not going over all the reflexes you still need to alternate between both feet. Each area represents an organ which may be paired and found on both sides of the body. So if you miss out one foot you could be stimulating only half an organ.

Will I have any adverse reactions from R.R.

Depending on the health of the recipient, sometimes after a full reflexology treatment, the body reacts in an attempt to rid itself of toxins, and consequently the eliminating systems of the body, may become more active. This can take the form of a more frequent need to pass urine, a rash, or the symptoms of a cold. This could happen in your first R.R. session, but it is very mild.

Zone Therapy Guide

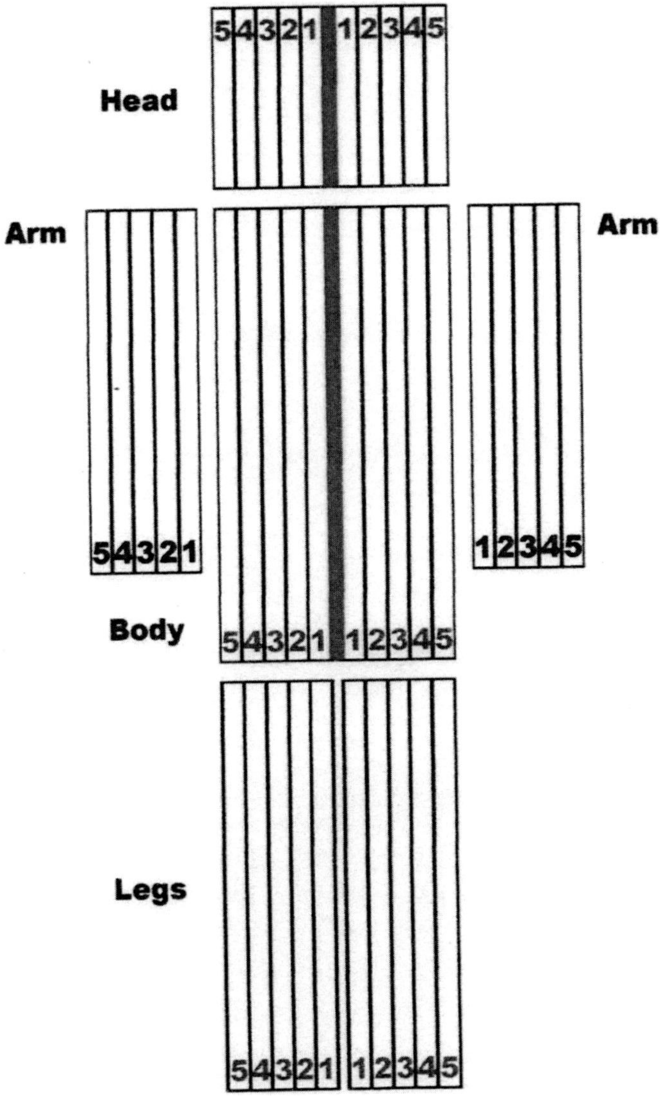

The Zone Theory

Dr Fitzgerald worked on the theory that the body could be divided into five zones on either side of a medial line. The ten zones ending in the fingers and toes as shown in the diagram. His theory consisted of the idea that the reflexes in the feet corresponded to the glands and organs in the body. This link was seen by the Doctor as the ten imaginary longitudinal lines each encompassing a zone. The zones run the length of the body, from the top of the head to the end of the toes. The reflexologist must be knowledgeable about both the zones and the parts of the body associated within them.

Most practitioners work mainly on the feet, although energy channels are thought to end in both the hands and feet. Doreen Bayly, founder of the Bayly school of reflexology assumed that the right foot is related to the right side of the body, and the left foot to the left side, which is illustrated on her particular chart. Although it must be remembered there is an exception to the rule. The right half of the brain controls the left side of the body, whilst the left half controls the right. A reflexologist needs to bear the exception in mind, for instance, when treating a stroke victim, who could be paralysed on one side of the body.

If the soles of the feet, side by side, are imagined as corresponding to the body then we can visualise the head being at the top. In order to view the body image being on the feet in a correct location we can use the guidelines suggested by the German reflexologist Hanne Marquardt. She put forward the idea that four imaginary transverse lines to the body should be used as further guidelines for the reflexologist.

Hanne Marquardt charted these four lateral lines as follows:

1. The shoulder line below the base of the toes. Of course anatomically the area is situated below the head and neck.

2. The diaphragm line just below the ball of the foot. On the body it separates the chest cavity from the abdominal cavity.

3. The waistline across the middle of the foot in the centre of the arch. The slender part of the body between the ribs and hips.

4. The pelvic line just above the heel. On the body it is the shape of a bony basin built into the bottom of the spine

By using these imaginary lines it makes it easier to place the various reflex points on the feet to map out a corresponding area on the body. In doing this it must be considered that internal organs overlap each other therefore the areas on the feet relating to them will overlap as well. Consequently this can be difficult to place on a foot chart therefore we have to have an image on the foot in a three-dimensional way which will represent a three dimensional body.

Cross-references can be found between shoulder and hip, elbow and knee, or hand and foot. When pain is felt at a distance from its point of origin, it is called "referred pain". In this case the reflexologist must be aware of various cross-references, if he/she is to treat correctly.

It may be that a "channel of energy", along the lines, joins organs in its path, but the lines must not be seen as veins, arteries, or nerve pathways. The professional practitioner believes that energy flows through each zone and when the energy is blocked by congestion, all kinds of illness can occur. Therefore reflexology is concerned with treating reflex points in order to stimulate the energy flow and by doing so helping the body to heal itself. If the circulation can be improved there is no doubt that it will influence the body to eliminate harmful toxins and waste deposits.

R.R. concentrates on relaxing tension and helping the body find its own equilibrium. This aspect will be dealt with in a later section.

Chapter Three

Reflexes on the feet in relation to the body

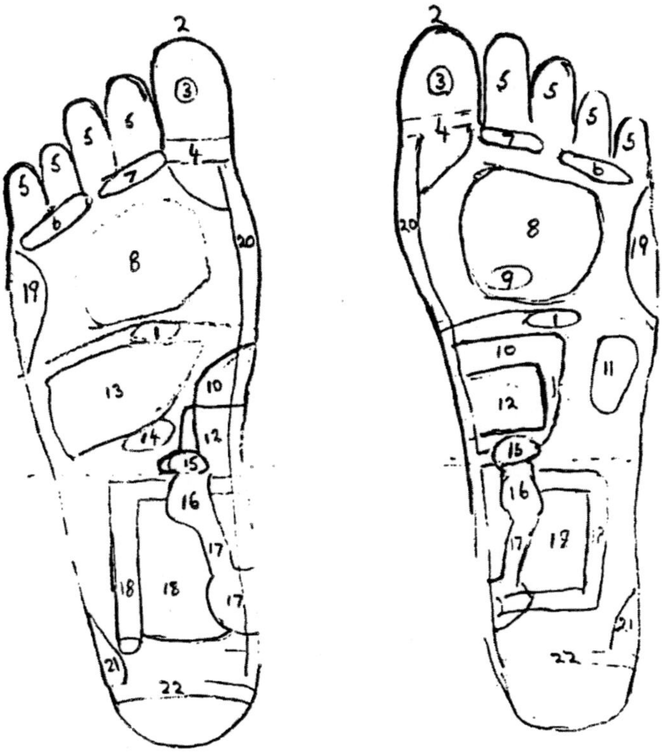

1 Solar plexus and diaphragm

2 Brain

3 Pituitary gland

4.Thyroid and parathyroid gland

5 Sinuses

6 Ears

7 Eyes

8 Lungs

9 Heart(left foot only)

10 Stomach

11 Spleen (left foot only)

12 Pancreas

13 Liver (right foot only)

14 Gall bladder (right foot only)

15 Adrenal gland

16 Kidney

17 Bladder, ureter and urethra

18 Intestines

19 Arm and shoulder

20 Spine

21 Hip, thigh and leg

Top of foot

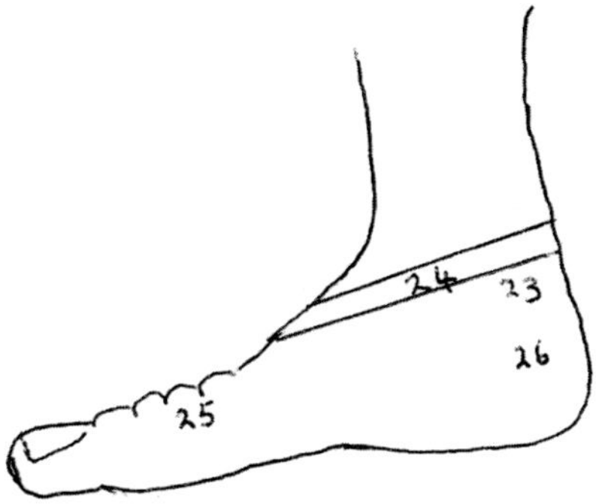

22. Sciatic nerve
23. Ovaries and testicles
24. Lymphatic system
25. Breasts
26. Uterus and prostate gland

There are some different versions of the 'foot map' in various schools of reflexology and the chart does not represent any particular school. Unlike most charts, I have placed the solar plexus and diaphragm at number one, in order to emphasise its relevance to R.R.

Reflex Areas on the Hands

Left Hand **Right Hand**

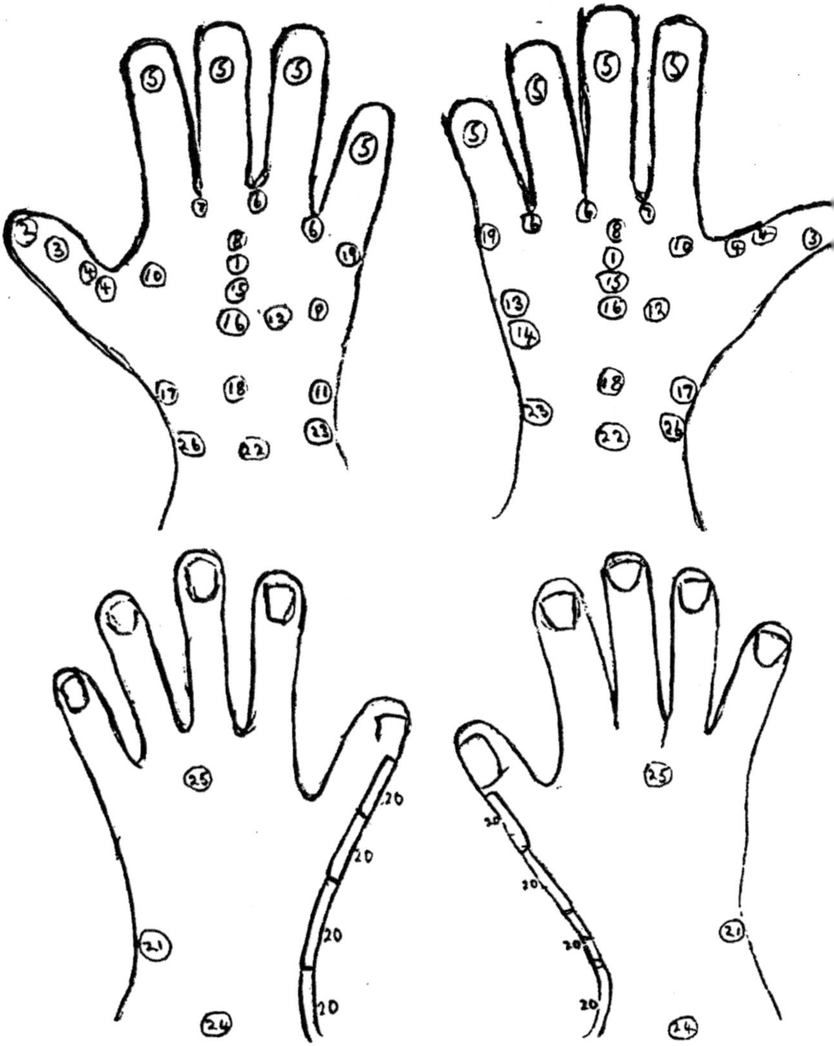

Found on Palm and Back of hands

1. Solar plexus and diaphragm(both hands)
2. Brain (both hands)
2. Pituitary gland (both hands)
3. Thyroid and parathyroid gland (both hands)
4. Sinuses (both hands)
5. Ear (both hands)
6. Eye (both hands)
7. Lung (both hands)
8. Heart (left hand only)
9. Stomach (both hands)
10. Spleen (left hand only)
11. Pancreas (both hands)
12. Liver (right hand only)
13. Gall bladder(right hand only)
14. Adrenal gland(both hands)
15. Kidney (both hands)
16. Bladder, Ureter, and Urethra(both hands)
17. Intestine (both hands)
18. Arm and Shoulder (both hands)
19. Spine (both hands)
20. Hip, Thigh, and leg (both hands)

21. Sciatic nerve (both hands)
22. Ovary and testicle (both hands)
23. Lymphatic system (both hands)
24. Breast (both hands)
25. Uterus and Prostate (both hands)

R.R. And the Hands

In my experience of giving reflexology, I have found that using it on the hands does not give the same relaxation compared to working on the feet. The reason could be a difference in sensitivity. Feet are well protected throughout one's life, by stockings and shoes, whereas hands are exposed to weather and all kinds of conditions at work and leisure. However in some cases a person may not be able to work on the feet or wish to have someone treat their feet. In this case, they may consider working the hand reflexes, and in so doing ought to be aware of the following.

Method used on the Hands

The professional reflexologist compares the hands to an electrical component, in which the right hand palm is positive, and the left hand palm is negative. Further than this it is considered that the right hand has a stimulating potential while the left has a soothing effect. The backs of the hands are seen as opposite to the palms, so the right is negative and the left positive. Therefore, a reflexologist would use the pressure points on the right hand to renew energy and the reflexes on the left hand to relieve pain. Similar to the foot; the right hand is for the right half of the body; and the left hand for the left half of the body.

When treating the hands it is important to be aware that the anatomical make-up is different from the foot. The reflexes are closer together and more immersed into the palm than reflexes found on the foot. Consequently, not as clearly defined, because they take up less area, making them more difficult to detect. Therefore, you should develop a comfortable technique for using your thumbs and fingers which can be used in much the same way as working on the feet.

The thumb is more appropriate for the palm area, whilst the fingers are best used as leverage on the top of the hand. Although if you work on the areas between the fingers, on the back of the hand, it is easier if the thumb is used for leverage on the palm whilst your index finger is used on the pressure points. Remember that in the case of self-help, you are only aiming to cover a limited number of pressure points and you may wish to modify the technique of how you use fingers and thumbs. One person told me she preferred making a rotation movement with the fingers; while another said he used a pumping action on the palm area and a stroking action on the finger areas. Do not work on any area that is inflamed or showing other apparent problems.

As with the feet, do not use the hand method to treat an unknown illness, if you are feeling ill it is best to let a competent doctor decide what you are suffering from. It is also foolhardy to ignore modern scientific techniques available to treat stress. R.R. does not decry medicine it aims to work with it.

Get your Act together

Most books about reflexology give half the books space over to a discussion about anatomy and physiology. If you wish to study for a professional qualification to practice then an intensive study of both subjects is necessary. There are many books giving detailed information about how the body works so it is not the intention of this book to reproduce such knowledge.

However, in my lectures I constantly use the technical term "homeostasis", which is defined in the dictionary as a strong state of balance. For the purposes of teaching R.R. I ask my students to imagine homeostasis as being the middle ground between a stressed condition and a relaxed condition. They are asked to visualise homeostasis counteracting the effects of stress.

In order to prevent illness the body must be in a state of homeostasis. The therapy can play a part in bringing the mind and body back into balance by concentrating on achieving relaxation.

The Balancing Act

Although the various structures and fluids of the body are different superficially, in reality they are constructed from the same basic unit, namely the cell. The process by which the cell utilizes the nutritional elements brought to it by the blood stream is a result of the digestion and absorption of food, known as metabolism. It is by means of this metabolic process that food we eat is transformed into living tissue.

The constant building up and breaking down of tissue produces unwanted waste products which must be removed from the body to prevent a general clogging of the whole system. If the body's attempt to rid itself of the debris referred to is prevented, the waste materials, acid in character, are put back into the tissues. When this happens, they can find refuge in the inner parts of the body, around the joints and nerve sheaths, with the result that uric-acid diseases appear, such as rheumatism, gout, arthritis, and sciatica. It is also may accumulate in the lungs or other organs including the heart.

In order to understand healthy cell metabolism (not to be confused with unwise food habits) we need to look first at the system of elimination. Acid waste products are formed which are neutralized by the alkaline mineral salts in the cell, in the presence of water and oxygen, the neutralized product is carried away by the blood and lymph. It is this process, which we can call elimination.

The body achieves regular cleansing by using four channels, chiefly the lymph nodes, kidneys, colon, and the skin. It is very important health wise that these channels remain free from blockage to avoid a build-up of toxins.

If toxins are allowed to accumulate, the body will lose its natural state of balance and the organs are weakened. This can be by way of a diminished blood flow to the organs, which then slows down the oxygen, and nutrients to the cells. The cells can then die and consequently organs and glands are unable to function correctly making it difficult to maintain their balancing effect.

The cause of unhealthy cell metabolism is not all due to a faulty diet. Not least among other factors is stress that can lead to enervation and nervous exhaustion.

Relaxation Contributes Towards Healthy cell Metabolism.

The main purpose of R.R. is to help the mind and body regain Homeostasis, or balance, through relaxation. If the body is constantly in a state of tension, natural bodily processes are interfered with. For the body to be in a good state of equilibrium it needs to be free from damaging tensions which prevent it from returning to a well-balanced condition. R.R. together with reflexology seeks to give the individual beneficial therapy to aid the body use its natural process in restoring itself.

It can accomplish this in the following ways. By bringing a state of relaxation to the body, it combats muscular contraction. If prolonged tension causes muscles to remain in a state of contraction, organs and glands become tight, resulting in restriction from functioning properly.

As our musculature relaxes not only do we become more relaxed physically but also mentally and emotionally. An environment is created whereby newly formed cells are able to rejuvenate the body under advantageous conditions.

The therapy in reducing stress and tension allows a more efficient blood flow that helps the cardiovascular system carry oxygen and nutrients unimpeded to the cells. When this takes place the waste products of metabolism, and toxins are removed by the free flow of blood. If the body stays in a tense rigidity which restricts mobility, then potentially toxic matter can eventually gather in the lymphatic vessels.

We must be aware of the necessity for cells to be nurtured so that they are able to restore themselves under the best provisions. Reflexology is a tool that can give the individual a means to assist the body in having a resiliency for correct functioning, and by so doing, contributing towards a state of balance.

The Mission Statement

To be Successful R.R. must give R.R. (Relaxation Response)

Before we begin to use the technique, we need to be quite sure what our aim is. It is to gain a 'relaxation response.' The opposite of a highly tensed up state now commonly referred to as the 'fight or flight' stress condition.

In order to deal with a stressful situation the sympathetic nervous system takes over and hormones are released. The metabolic rate is increased. There is a quickened heart rate, faster breathing, and muscles tense. To compensate the condition the parasympathetic counterpart should regenerate the body's energies. The problem arises when the highly stressed up state goes on for too long without relief. Then a kind of "overdrive" situation is created and we have a build-up of harmful stress. Unless we discharge the stress and relax, chronic tension takes over.

The idea behind R.R. is to assist the body and mind experience a 'relaxation response' in a prolonged period of relaxation. Recipients have told me that until they experienced deep relaxation they had no idea of what tension really was. Some people fall asleep quite often. If a sense of being relaxed and energised is not present, then full benefits from the session have not taken place.

Chapter Four

Preparing the feet For Reflex-Relaxology

In order to counteract the disadvantage of not having a full reflexology treatment you should give yourself the following special foot massage. Find a comfortable position so you can place hands on feet without any strain. To achieve this you may find any of the following best, sitting on a floor, chair, bed, or whatever suits you.

You may need to bathe your feet or wipe them with a warm sponge. Then examine them carefully for any calluses, sores, corns, cuts, or anything that could cause irritation, if touched. I often find it necessary to advice a recipient that they should have chiropody treatment before reflexology. Athlete's foot seems very common, but it is easily preventable if the feet are always thoroughly cleaned particularly between the toes. Good foot hygiene will not allow the fungus causing Athlete's foot to thrive.

When you are satisfied there is no irritation on your feet you are ready for the next step. Use a rotary circular motion with the pads of your fingers for this foot massage

Begin on the bottom of the feet, by massaging the soles. Then gradually and gently work up the sides and ankles, still using the circular method. The pressure you are using will depend upon the reaction you are receiving. If it is a feeling of soreness or pain, then you are perhaps being too vigorous, or you have a problem from an old injury.

Circulation in the feet

This careful foot massage will not only prepare the feet for R.R. but can bring vitality to a sluggish circulation which may need to be speeded up. Because the feet are farthest from the heart circulation is often at its weakest point in the feet. The heart has to drive the blood down then the blood must flow against gravity to return to the heart.

If our life-style is not governed by common sense and correct nutrition that allows the function of good mastication, digestion, assimilation, and elimination, then we are left with a retention and accumulation of a toxic residue. This build-up in the body results in gravity forcing acid crystals downward until they become deposited in the feet During the massage and R.R. treatment you may become aware of these crystalline deposits which can be carefully massaged out by using either your thumb or the pads of your fingers for pressure.

Using the Technique

Before giving or receiving reflex-relaxology, it is important to remember the therapy is complementary to orthodox medicine and should not be used in place of such. It is not a medical treatment. The professional reflexologist does not practice medicine or diagnose illness. Also, until more research has been undertaken it may not be wise to treat some conditions.

Reflexology is probably the safest of all the complementary therapies but when I was training, it was considered wrong to treat anyone who had a thrombosis or embolism in case a blood clot moved. We were instructed not to treat a person who had inflammation of the venous and lymphatic systems, heart condition and anything where surgery was needed. The list also included high temperature sickness, fungal infection, or other infectious illness.

Since then there is a lot of disagreement and confusion about what reflexology should not treat. It is best to be aware of the following problems.

It may not be appropriate treatment for diabetics in some cases.

A pacemaker on a person has been known to move when the chest area reflex on the left foot received pressure.

If the gall bladder and liver reflexes on someone ill with renal (kidney) calculi are used it could move the stones.

There is much argument about it being used during pregnancy in the first trimester.

Despite the fact of nine studies demonstrating its benefit for mental health, it is thought wrong to use it on persons who are psychotic, taking psychoactive drugs, in depressive and manic states, or suffering from clinical depression.

Therefore, it is wise not to treat the conditions mentioned, or any other, until advice and permission has been given from the recipients medical consultant that reflexology will do no harm.

Also, remember self-treatment will never give you the amount of relaxation that treatment from a reflexologist can give. Mainly because there can never be the same healing elements involved. In giving yourself R.R., you are acting as recipient and therapist so you should see it as contributing to a professional reflexology session and not a complete treatment.

Most reflexologists use the thumb to give pressure, but it may be difficult to use this method on oneself, and you may find the fingers are more comfortable to use. To begin with, try using the thumb or finger to make circular and rocking motions as you move from one reflex to another. As you become more proficient in using the technique, become aware of gaining an intuitive approach. Such an approach depends upon the individual's response to how much pressure and refinements of movement they use.

Be careful not to overdo time spent on a reflex; it could over stimulate certain areas instead of giving balance in the body. When first starting, ten minutes is all you need, consisting of a few seconds spent on each area and giving a few light pressures to the reflex points.

Above all, be aware that the aim is to give you relief from tension. The whole method should be carried out in a relaxed and calm state.

Using the Thumb

Thumb Pressure

Thumb pressure simply means bending the first joint of the thumb and using it in a caterpillar sequence along the specific areas you wish to treat. Gradually, with a little practice you will be able to give the thumb a rocking effect from the top of the thumb to the bottom.

This technique can be difficult to achieve at first, and may need a lot of practice. Be careful that you do not slip from the correct position and cause the thumbnail to dig into the skin. Try to become skilled in gaining a firm, but comfortable pressure.

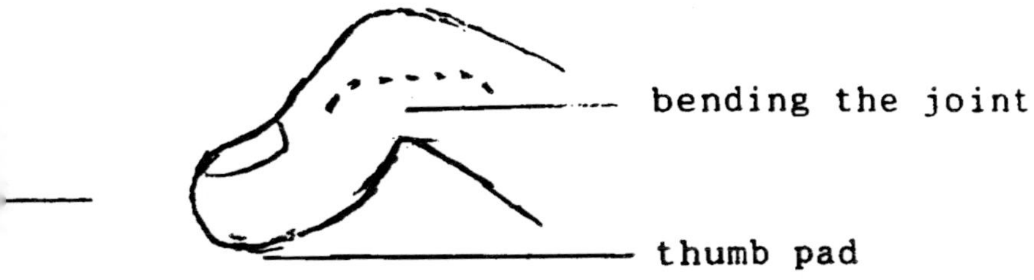

Using the Fingers

Finger Pressure

This is very similar to using the_thumb in the way described. The first joint of the finger is given a slight rocking motion from the finger top to the bottom of the finger pad. Without some practice, it may be difficult to bend the joint. You can overcome this by practicing on the top of your hand which will give you an idea of how hard you are pressing. Gradually you will find the fingers losing their stiffness as you practice.

Remember in using R. R. you should not worry about any definite rules for using thumbs or fingers. The main criteria are to feel at ease and if that means creating your own method it is compatible with the idea of R. R.

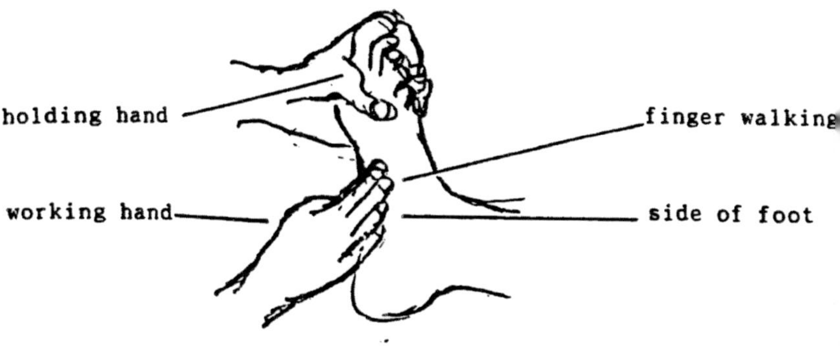

R.R. Chart

This chart shows the reflex areas you should work on for reflex-relaxology. For a full reflexology treatment use the chart at the beginning of the book.

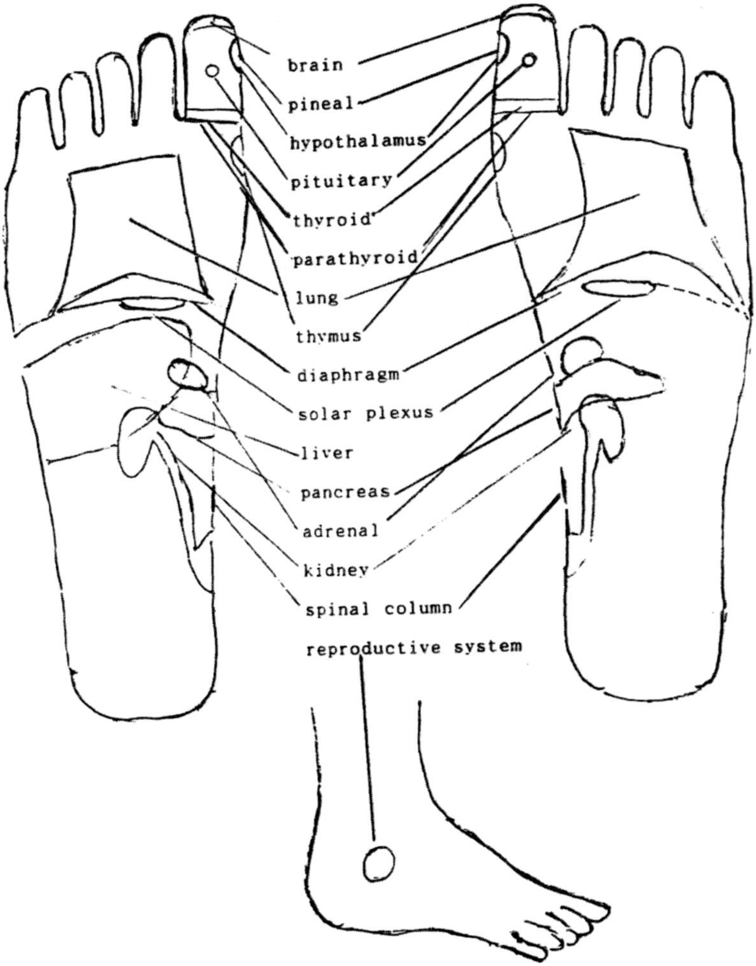

The R.R. Pressure Points

1. Solar plexus and diaphragm reflexes
2. Brain reflexes
3. Spine reflexes
4. Pituitary gland reflexes
5. Adrenal glands reflexes
6. Thyroid/parathyroid glands reflexes
7. Lung reflexes
9. Kidney reflexes
10. Reproductive gland reflexes

The following explains the relevance of the particular reflex, where to find it, and a comfortable way to apply the pressure. Begin and end with gentle pressure on the solar plexus and diaphragm reflexes.

Memory reference for the sixteen reflex points used in reflex- relaxology.

solar plexus

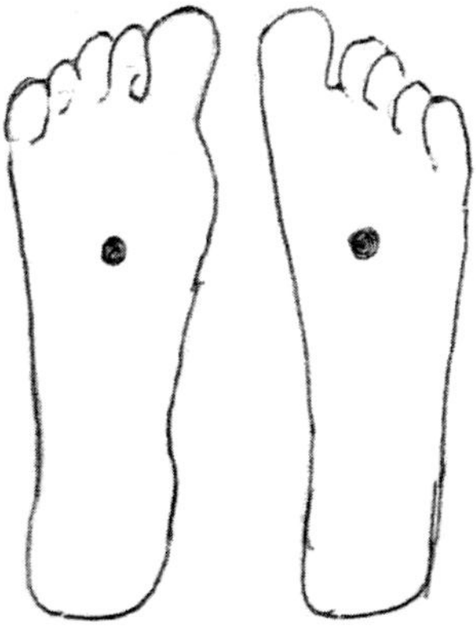

diaphragm

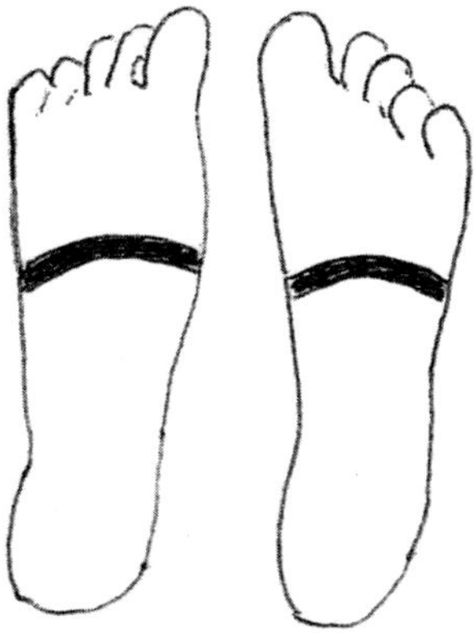

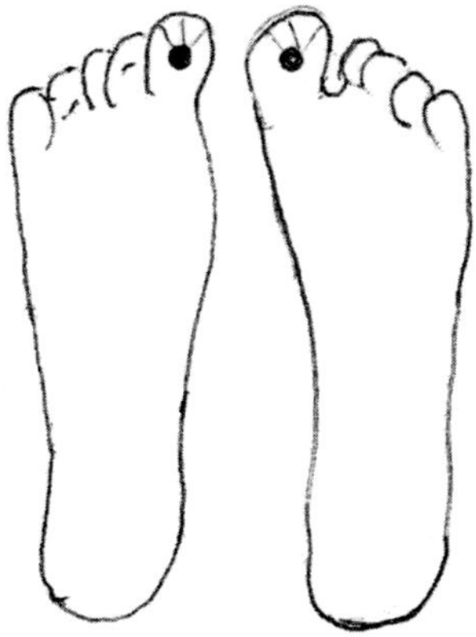

brain

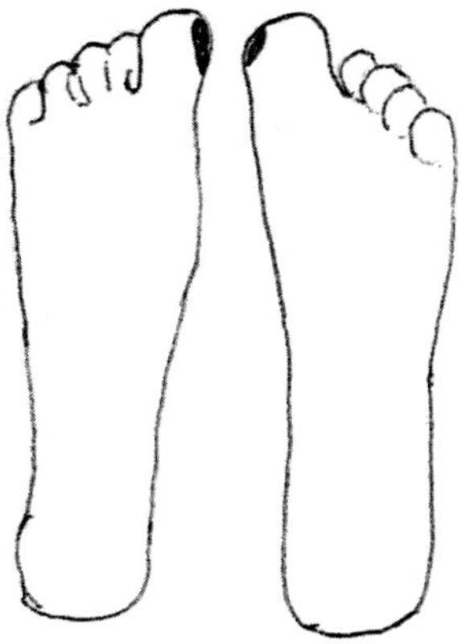

pineal

hypothalamus

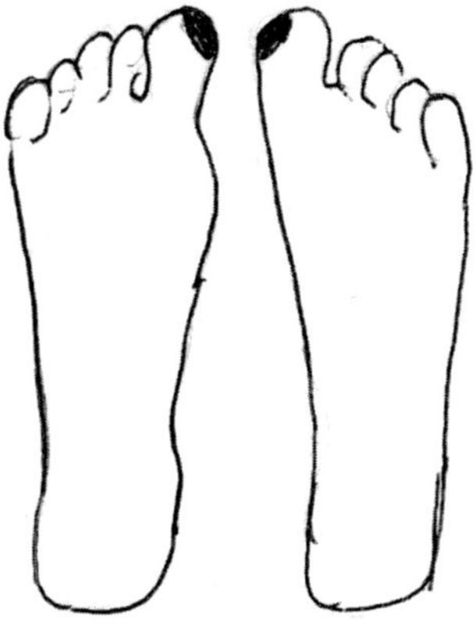

pituitary

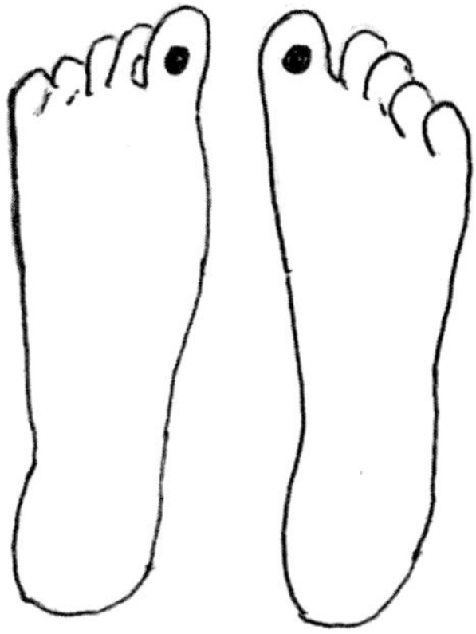

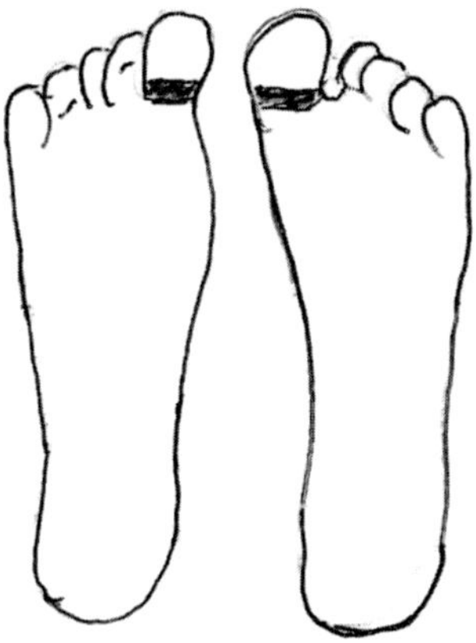

parathyroid

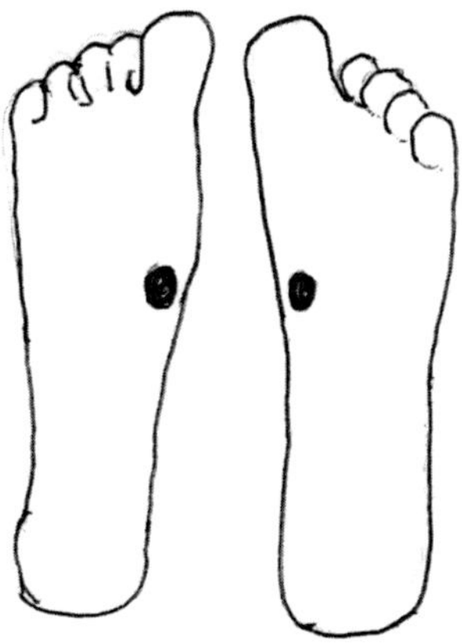

adrenal

thyroid

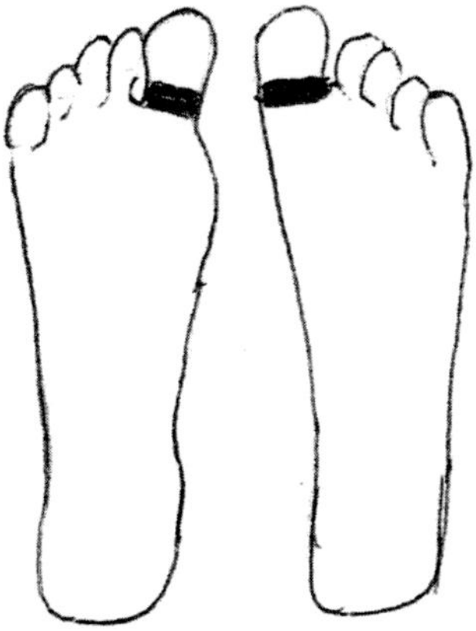

thymus

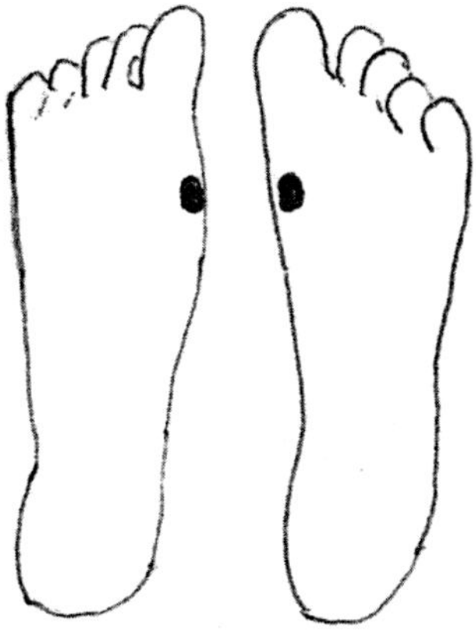

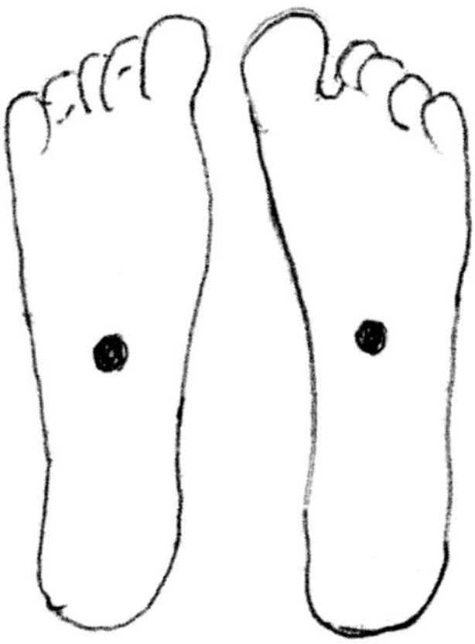

kidney

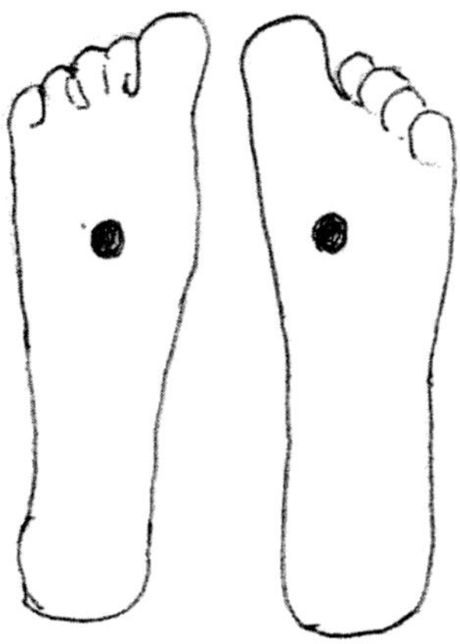

liver

pancreas

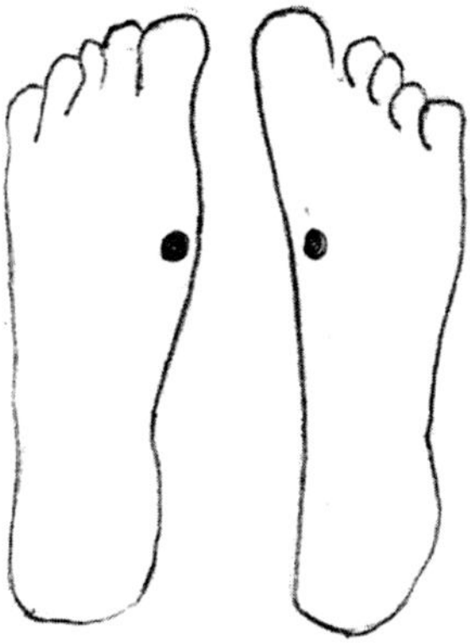

lung

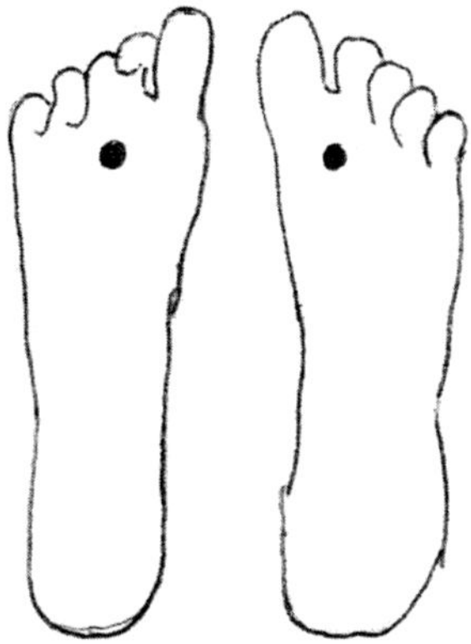

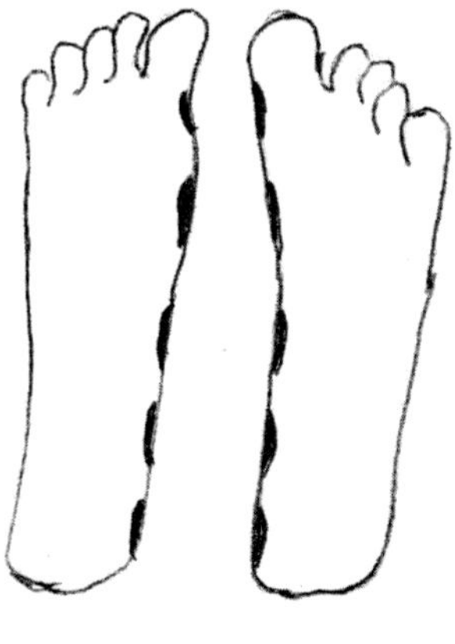

spine

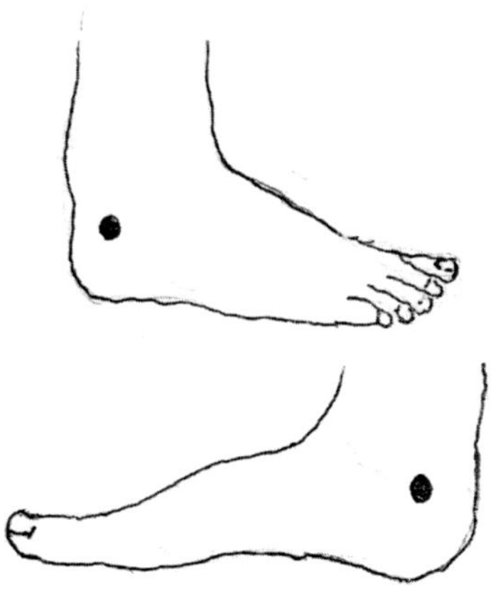

reproductive

Solar Plexus

Relevance.

The solar plexus is number one in the R.R. programme. It is a network of nerves connected to all parts of the body. Pressure on this area can relax the whole nervous system.

Reflex-area.

On both feet between the big toe and the second toe. On the sole of the foot imagine a line extending across the lower area of the ball of the big toe and the ball of each foot. In the hands the reflex is found in the area between thumb and second finger across the palm of the hand.

Application.

For ones own purposes the position of the hands in holding the feet is not important. Feeling comfortable is what matters. The aim is to feel relaxed not to make further tension of any kind. Leave the various foot holding techniques to the professional reflexologist. I suggest gentle pressure of thumb or fingers in a circular motion to cover the area. Always include this pressure point in your self-treatment plan.

Diaphragm

Relevance.

An excellent reflex to work in releasing tension. It is the main muscle used for good breathing, and any imbalance in this area can cause breathing problems.

Reflex-area.

The diaphragm reflexes are found in both feet and hands. On the sole of the foot follow an imaginary line from the bottom area of the big toe across the ball of each foot. The solar plexus is found on the same level.

In the hands the reflex is found in the area between thumb and second finger across the palm of the hand.

Application.

A reflexologist would use a thumb walking technique for this area, which is fine, if you can manage to bend your thumb whilst holding your foot with your free hand. If not try holding back your toes with one hand and using the other hand, either fingers or thumb, in a gentle rotating massage combining finger or thumb pressure.

Brain

Relevance.

It is important to remember that in the central nervous system where the brain plays a considerable part in the function of communication to all parts of the body that here we have the exception to the reflexology zonal concept. In this case the right half of the brain controls the left side of the body and the left half of the brain controls the right side of the body. Unlike the zone concept of the right foot representing the right side of the body and the left foot the left side.

Awareness of the exception is necessary when treating any disorders of the nervous system, or brain, and pressure points on the correct parts of the foot, on the opposite side from the stress is crucial.

Reflex- area.

The brain and head reflexes are found in the big toes and the thumbs. The top of the brain and top of the head are situated in the pads of the big toes and in the pads of the thumbs.

Application.

The main area to concentrate on is the tips and pads of the toes. Not just the big toes but all the toes should be worked on. Use a rolling motion with the index finger of one hand whilst the free hand holds the toe steady.

Pineal Gland

Relevance

Although the function of this gland is not fully understood it should not be left out as it is thought to have a connection with a persons moods. New knowledge suggests it may regulate natural variations in the body's rhythms over a 24-hour interval. These two functions make it a part of the programme.

Reflex-area.

Located on top of the big toe at the inner side of both feet. On the hands it is found near the top of the thumb on the pad near to the pituitary reflex.

Application.

Use the holding hand to support the big toe and gently rotate the corner of the thumb over the point. If this does not feel comfortable then use the index finger in the same way.

Hypothalamus

Relevance.

The hypothalamus is a special area of grey matter situated in the forebrain. It is of particular importance in R.R. because it controls secretions from the pituitary gland, and is linked to the autonomic nervous system. Consequently the gland controls our emotions and body temperature.

Reflex-area.

It has the same reflex point as the pineal, found near the pituitary reflex on the inner side and top of the big toes. Remember that each big toe has reflex areas for; the pituitary, pineal, hypothalamus, brain, temples, upper and lower jaw, gums, teeth, throat, thyroid/parathyroid, and the seven cervical vertebra. The reflex points can also be found near the centre of the pads of both thumbs

Application.

Treat this area before working the pituitary reflex because of the link in controlling secretions. Use a very gentle massage with either thumb or finger, for a few seconds only, then press the reflex, hold for a few seconds and release slowly.

Pituitary Gland

Relevance.

The pituitary gland regulates all the other glands involved in metabolism (the rate at which cells work). Correct pressure to this point can help to maintain your emotional balance.

Reflex-area.

Centre of the big toe on both feet and centre of the thumb found on both hands.

Application.

Best to use one hand for leverage, which will prevent painful bending of the toe. The corner of the thumb on the working hand is probably the most effective for treating this point.

Parathyroid Glands

Relevance.

These four small glands located within the thyroid are very important in keeping a normal metabolic balance of the body.

The parathyroids through their hormones control the level of calcium and phosphorous in the blood. Their main relevance to relaxation is because the level of calcium in the blood is involved in the actions of the nerves.

Reflex- area.

Just above the neckline at the base of the big toe in both feet, and in a similar position on the thumbs of both hands.

Application

Support the big toe with the holding hand and let the Fingers of the working hand rest on those of the holding hand. Then thumb walk so that you cover the whole area a few times, changing hands if necessary.

Adrenal glands

Relevance.

These glands are very instrumental in helping the Body cope with stress. The adrenalin is often referred to as the "fight or flight" hormone, but it is also concerned with helping the body cope with inflammatory problems.

Reflex-area.

The reflexes are situated in the same area as that of the kidneys but are not related. Find them between the waistline and the diaphragm line, on the inside near the protruding tendon. Located in both palms of the hands near the inside of the pad at the base of the thumb.

Application.

If you are working on your own feet then it may be more comfortable to use your fingers in a rotating manner but a reflexologist is more likely to use the thumb walk. Because of the proximity of the adrenal reflexes to those of the kidney, be careful not to over-stimulate the kidney reflex by spending too long on this area.

Thyroid

Relevance.

This gland his very important in helping the body return to calmness and regulating body temperature. It controls the metabolism that affects our energy levels, and the reflex can be worked to help regulate body functions. Both the thyroid and the parathyroid gland reflexes can be instrumental in encouraging muscle tension back into balance.

Reflex-area.

Found above the neck area of the big toe. This is at the bottom near the sole of the foot. It is the part of the top half of the ball of the big toe or thumb and is found in both the right and left feet or hands.

Application.

Use a holding hand on the toe to hold it in position for the free hand to work the reflex. Hold it firm but comfortable so that it will be stationary while your working hand is able to thumb walk over a large area for this reflex.

To remain comfortable and change the thumbs direction use alternate hands for holding and working.

Thymus Gland

Relevance.

Included in the R.R. programme mainly because of the dependence of T-lymphocytes (bone marrow cells) upon the presence of the thymus. The gland is also thought to play a part in the body's immune system particularly during childhood.

Reflex-area.

Found on both soles of the feet and situated on the medial half of the ball of the big toe In the palms of both hands on the ball of each thumb.

Application.

Use thumb pressure or you can massage with the fingers making a rotary movement. Massage the whole area from the diaphragm reflex to the bottom of the big toes.

Kidney

Relevance.

We should treat this area to clear poison wastes from the body and to help the kidneys keep correct blood pressure. If the kidneys malfunction it becomes difficult for proper elimination of the bodies waste products. By relaxing the body we help the elimination process to keep in good working order.

Reflex-area.

Found on both feet in the centre of the foot above and below the waist level guidelines and on the outside of the tendon. It is on both palms of the hands near the inside of the pad at the base of the thumb.

Application.

You will probably find using your thumb and fingers comfortable for this point but be aware of any tenderness, as hard pressure on this reflex will cause pain. Increase and decrease the pressure until you feel it is correct for you. Also be particularly careful not to overwork this reflex.

Liver

Relevance.

The liver is the largest organ in the body, situated mainly on the right side. It has over 500 functions but the two relevant ones to R.R. consist of the storage of glycogen that can be used to give the body an increased supply of energy, and the livers ability to detoxify the blood.

Reflex- area.

Found only on the right foot, situated in the sole, between the diaphragm and waist reflex area. It is also present in the palm of the right hand just below diaphragm level.

Application.

If you are working this area yourself the comfortable way is by using the fingers with the thumb resting on top of the foot. Use a gentle pressure, or a rotating movement covering the whole area. Also, as with the kidney reflex do not overwork.

Pancreas Gland

Relevance.

For proper digestion of food the pancreas must be working correctly. Diabetes can result from the gland not making enough insulin and thus failing to control sugar or glucose levels in the blood.

Reflex-area.

The area lies mainly on the left foot. Locate it from the waist guideline and then halfway to the diaphragm. On the right foot it is found a little below the waistline. On the palms it is near to the stomach reflex.

Application.

Thumb pressure is best for this location starting on the left foot and move across on to the right foot making sure the whole area is covered. Use a small caterpillar movement. It is usually a rather tender area so be extra careful with the amount of pressure used.

Lung

Relevance.

Working on the lung area helps to maintain the metabolic processes necessary to sustain and nourish the body. The pressure on this area of the feet helps to increase the bloods oxygen amount. The bloods oxygen level is important in the fight against stress.

Reflex- area.

Found at the base of the second, third, and fourth toes. On the hands the points are found in the pads at the base of the fingers. It should be remembered that also in this area is the breast and chest area.

Application.

The most comfortable way to treat yourself on the lung area is by using the whole pads of the fingers on one hand whilst grasping the top of the foot with the free hand. When I give a professional treatment I use the back of the fingers of the fist, not the knuckles, onto the soft area on the ball of the foot.

Spine

Relevance.

For our purposes we can think of the spine as part of a telephone system in which the central exchange in the brain has its branch exchanges in the spinal cord. Nerves from the spinal cord convey messages from the peripheral nerves of the body to the muscles and glands.

Reflex-area.

The spine area is located running along the inside edge of each foot from the base of the big toe down to approximately the heel. On the hands it is found on the medial borders of the thumbs.

Application.

To begin with use a whole palm stroking movement combined with slight pressure movements from the fingertips. Or any massage movement you find soothing. If you find certain areas sore you can then use either thumb or finger pressure.

Reproductive Glands

Relevance.

These glands must be included in our programme because hormones made by the reproductive organs affect every cell in the body. In fact these hormones play a part in our body's well being throughout the human life cycle.

Reflex-area.

The reflexes for these and related organs are situated close to the ankles on the inside of the feet. The ovary reflexes are found on the outer side of the foot. These reflexes can also be found on the arms near the wrists.

Application.

This part of the foot can be very sensitive and some difficulty can be found in working the correct point, so the pressure should be very light to start with, in case discomfort is felt. Experiment with thumb or finger pressure around the entire area.

Chapter Five

The R.R. Self-Monitoring Chart and basic Technique for Working on all the Areas.

The aim of the chart is to help you make an assessment of your technique in carrying out the R.R. application and its effectiveness. It can be used as a feedback that will monitor your progress. Furthermore it is a record of any problems encountered which can be discussed with a reflexologist. Write down in the comments section any benefits or otherwise.

Students who have undertaken this self-monitoring idea have remarked on how their comments have changed dramatically over a three-month period. See it as a record of how well you have learned the skill. You need only write a few words, such as, improved circulation, more energy, less tension. Used in this way the chart is a useful means of evaluating the effectiveness of R.R. both for yourself and others.

Unlike reflexology, which treats all kinds of conditions, R.R. is only concerned with relaxation therapy. However, it may well be that you find other benefits. For instance, the treatment may increase blood flow and loosen up muscles, thereby reducing the accumulation of lactic acid. This can be noted on your chart, under the heading of effectiveness.

There are six headings on the chart compiled to give you a simple uncomplicated means to monitor using the therapy. The following is an explanation of each heading.

Prepare Yourself

Find a comfortable position that gives you freedom to carry out the exercises without tensing up the body. Try to visualise and cultivate a calm feeling which you keep throughout the procedure.

Feet Evaluation

The condition of your feet can change very easily so use R.R. as a check-up time for observing any problems common to the feet. It is an opportunity to give proper nail care if needed. There are many disorders related to toenails and some complaints may mean a visit to a chiropodist.

Correct Pressure

Be aware of how much pressure is comfortable and take care not to overwork the reflex points. It will take experience to become skilful in using the pressure technique. At first you will have some trial and error.

Touch Quality

Do not underestimate the healing touch. The success of some chiropractics could be due to the development of the therapeutic use of their sense of touch. Seek constantly to improve your quality of touch, in combination with awareness that you are touching sensitive nerve endings in the feet.

Note Change

One definite change you should notice as you progress in giving yourself treatment is more skin pliability. In addition, dead cells exfoliated from the skins surface result in tone and texture improvement.

Effectiveness

After about three months of regular treatment a few times a week, you should be able to decide whether any benefits are apparent. If you are experiencing discomfort after treatment, it could be due to the release of waste products into the system. However if the discomfort is there after every session it may not be due to the therapy and you should seek medical advice. Very often agitation and tension is caused by a serious malfunction in the body needing a medical diagnosis. Such a state may have been caused by stress and then developed into a condition where relaxation will not make any difference.

The R.R. Self-Monitoring Chart

Description	Comments
Prepare Yourself	
Feet Evaluation	
Correct Pressure	
Touch Quality	
Note Changes	
Effectiveness	

Basic Techniques for Working on All the Areas

The previous sixteen reflex pressure points were those used in the R.R. therapy. The movements of the thumbs and fingers were explained in a way that could be comfortable for self- help. However reflexology is a fascinating subject and if you decide to train for qualification you should have some idea of how the professional reflexologist works. Also if you decide to have treatment it will give you knowledge of what he/she is doing.

The following movements described, and illustrated, are those personally used in my work as a reflexologist. I have found them to be the most efficient for the recipients needs. However, some reflexologists may use different variations. It is the recipient who will decide on which method is the best. Therefore if you practice this sequence of movements be fully aware of the effect your fingers and thumbs are having on your partner.

You must aim to give a sense of well-being. If the person is not receiving relief from tension then it doesn't matter how expert you become at using the following hand skills.

Relax the Feet first

Reflexologists treat all the reflexes on both feet, sometimes twice over, beginning usually with the right foot. Some believe that it is linked to the past, and so emotions must be released before present and future influences are met with in the left foot. I normally leave the preference to the recipient. However, we will begin the illustrations with the standard practice of beginning with the right foot. It is alright to first of all loosen up the feet by using the pre-R.R. technique before beginning to work on your partner's reflex points, I always begin a treatment by applying a gentle pressure to the solar plexus reflex area.

Solar Plexus

If you grip the top of the foot and squeeze, a depression will be evident on the sole of the foot at the centre of the diaphragm line (that is the middle part of the base of the ball of the foot. This is the solar plexus reflex.

Place your hands on both feet, as shown, and ask the subject to inhale slowly as you press on the point and exhale as you release pressure.

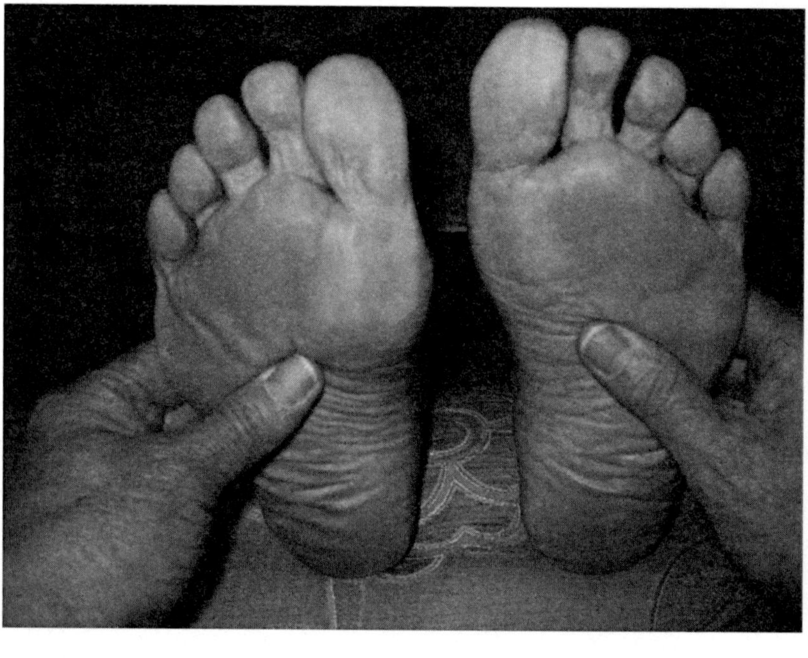

Diaphragm

The Diaphragm area is where the reflexologist gives particular attention to releasing tension. The location is more detectable if you gently pull the toes back with your left hand. Remember the solar plexus extends across the base of the ball of the foot. Thumb walk across the whole area working from the inside of the foot to the outside.

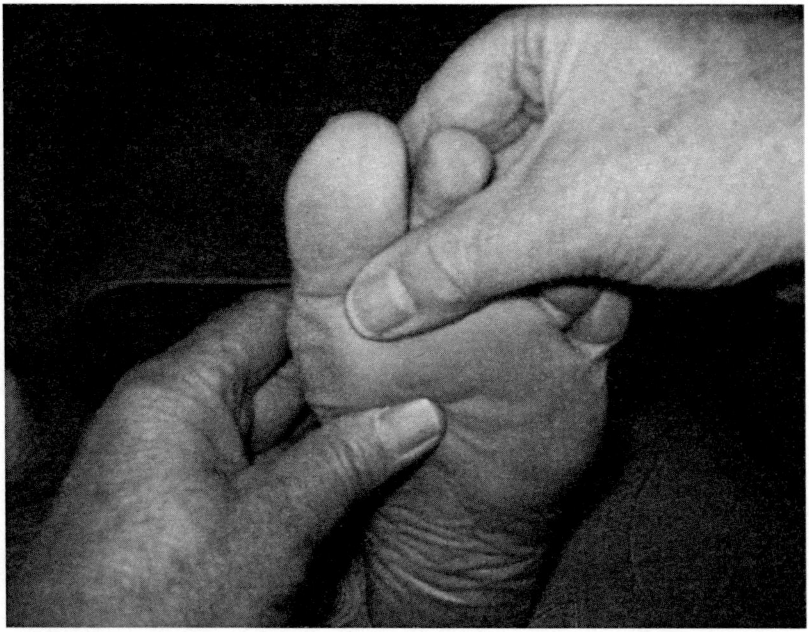

Brain Area

Make sure you have a firm grip with your holding hand at the back of the toes. Do not block the big toe with the holding hand. The toe must be free for the right thumb to give pressure by walking from the outer edge of the bottom of the toe up the outside, over the top and down the inside of the toe.

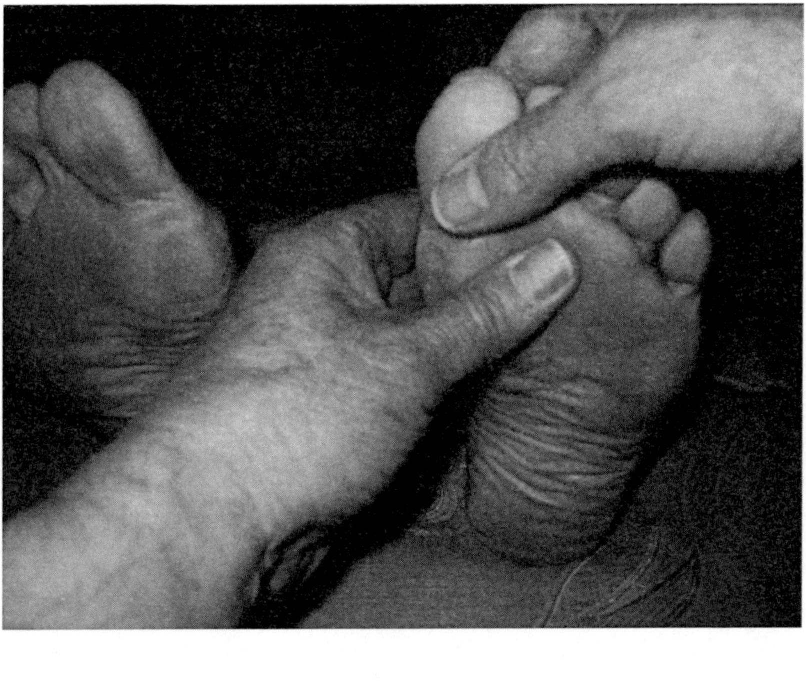

Pituitary Gland

Steady the toes with the left hand whilst finding approximately the middle part of the big toe. I find the 'hook in' technique best for this reflex point. The 'hook in' is usually needed when a point is to small for the walking technique. Use the four fingers on the working hand for leverage and apply pressure with the outside edge of the thumb on the reflex point. Be careful your nail does not dig in.

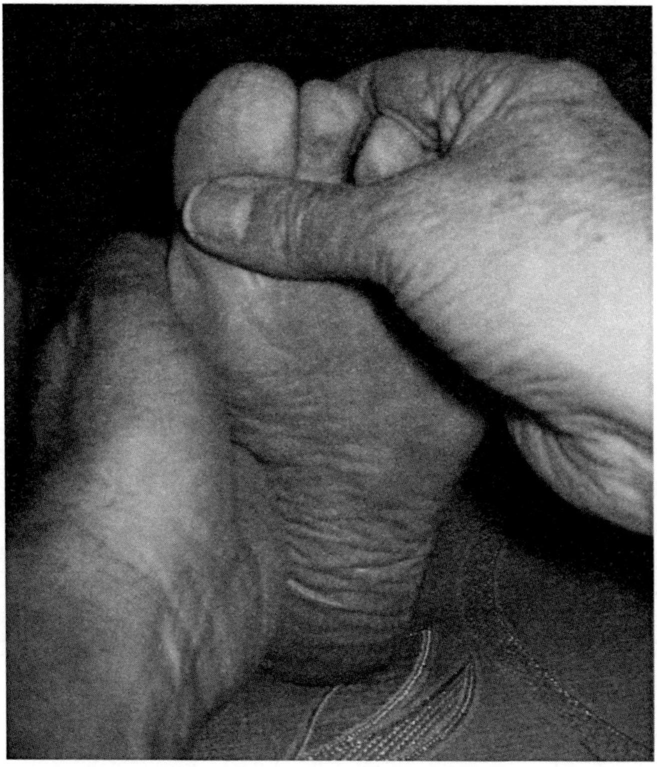

Face

Some reflexes overlap and the big toe contains many reflexes which include: pineal gland, pituitary gland, brain temples, teeth, the seven cervical (neck) vertebrae, sinuses, mastoid, tonsils, nose, and mouth. Hold the foot with the left hand, then with the fingers on top use the index finger to finger walk down the front of the big toe. Cover the area from the tip to the base. Caterpillar walk down the reflex a few times.

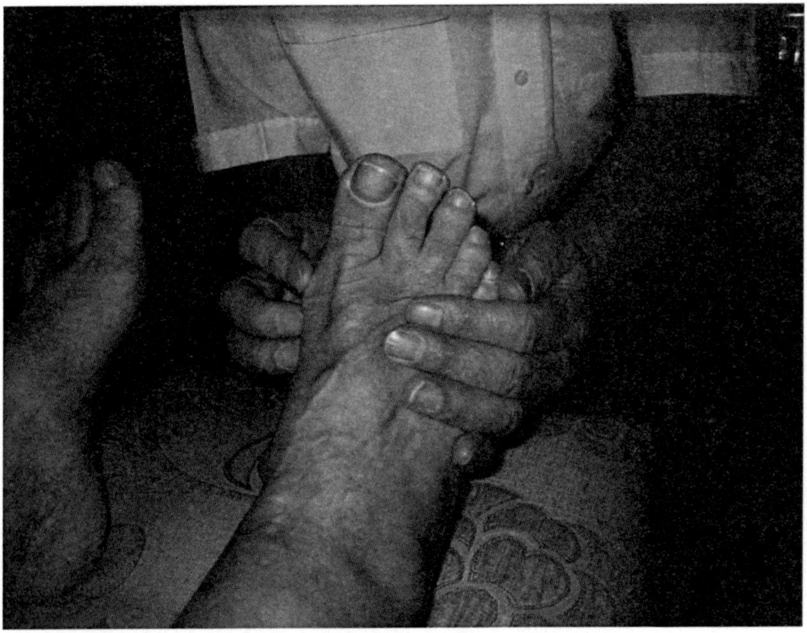

Neck

The working hand needs to hold the big toe between the thumb and index finger. Support the foot firmly while gently rotating the big toe first one way, then the other. The toe can be stiff and difficult to move so carefully loosen it by using the index finger to walk across the front base of the toe beginning from the outside to the inside.

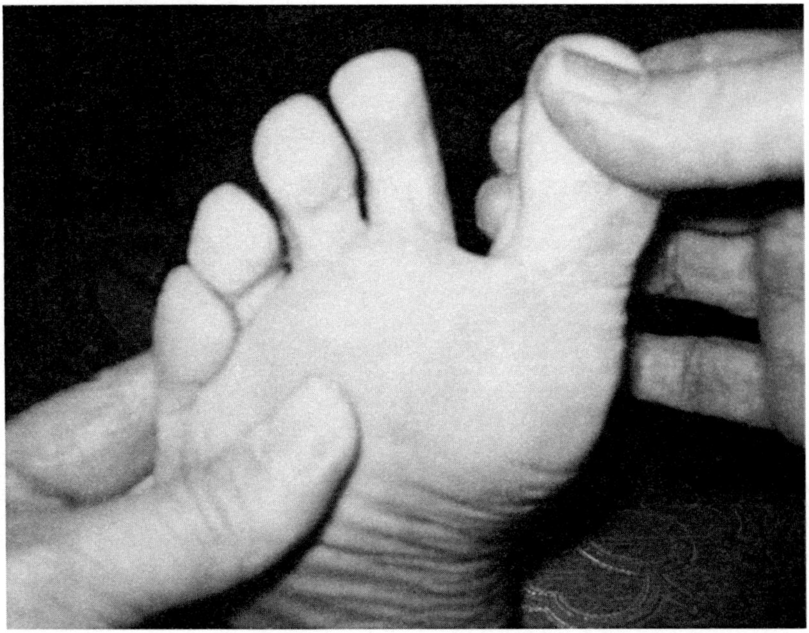

Thyroid/parathyroid

Support the big toe with the holding hand. Then use the thumb walking technique along the base of the big toe and the base of all the toes. This big toe area is important. It includes, pituitary, thyroid/parathyroid, 7th cervical and top of the head.

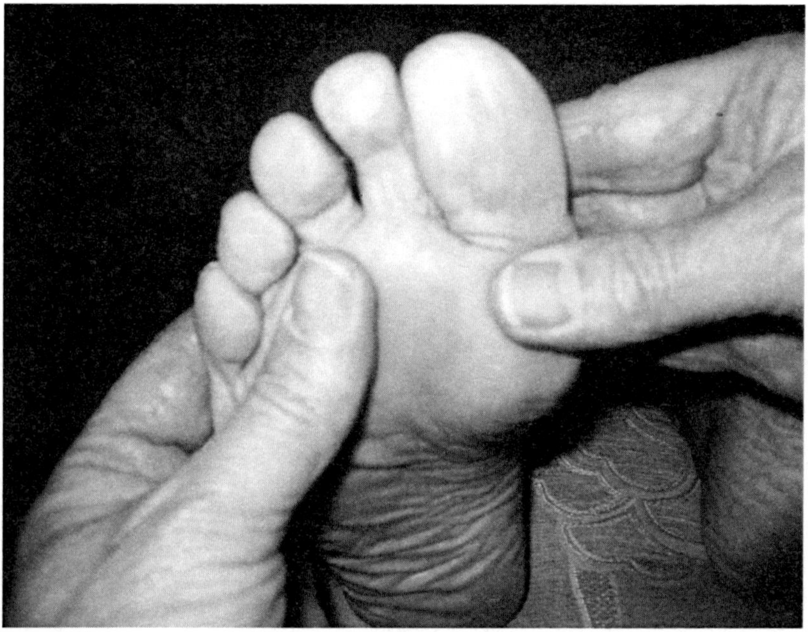

Sinuses

Whilst supporting the foot between the thumb and fingers of the left hand, use the right hand to thumb walk down the back, sides and top of the small toes. Work these areas two or three times.

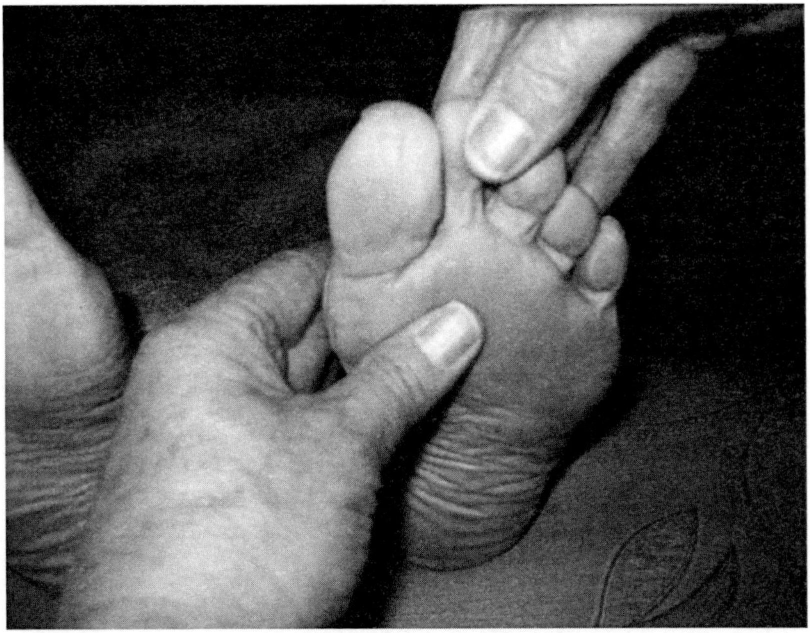

Ears/Eyes

For these areas the ridge at the base of the toes is worked. Carefully pull the toes back with the holding hand so the zones can be reached, but do not hold them back hard as this will make the skin tight.

Using the thumb walk across the ridge in both directions.

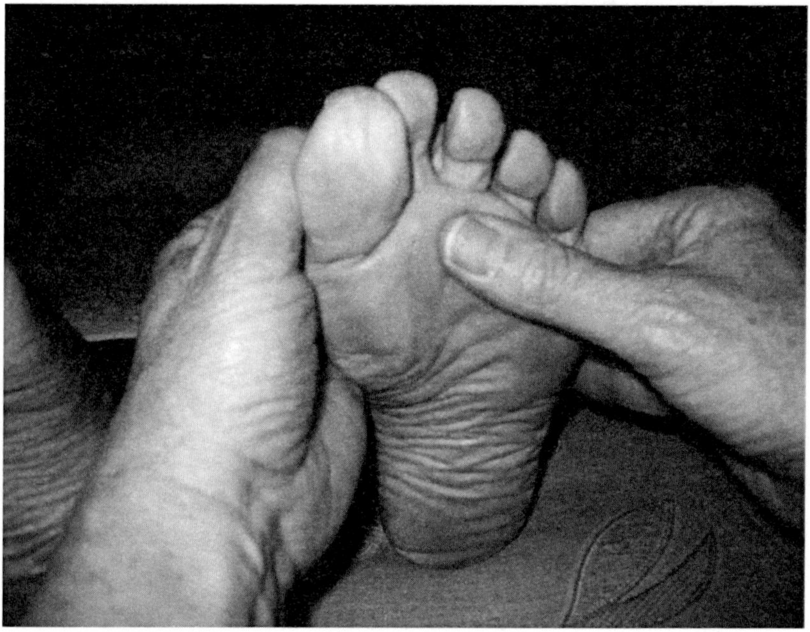

Chest/lung/breast

This zone consists of the area from the shoulder girdle line to the diaphragm line that covers the whole ball of the foot.

Hold the toes gently back. Then the right hand can be used to caterpillar walk, beginning from the base of the toes. Do it in vertical lines from the diaphragm to the shoulder girdle division on the sole of the foot. Finish by thumb walking the whole area.

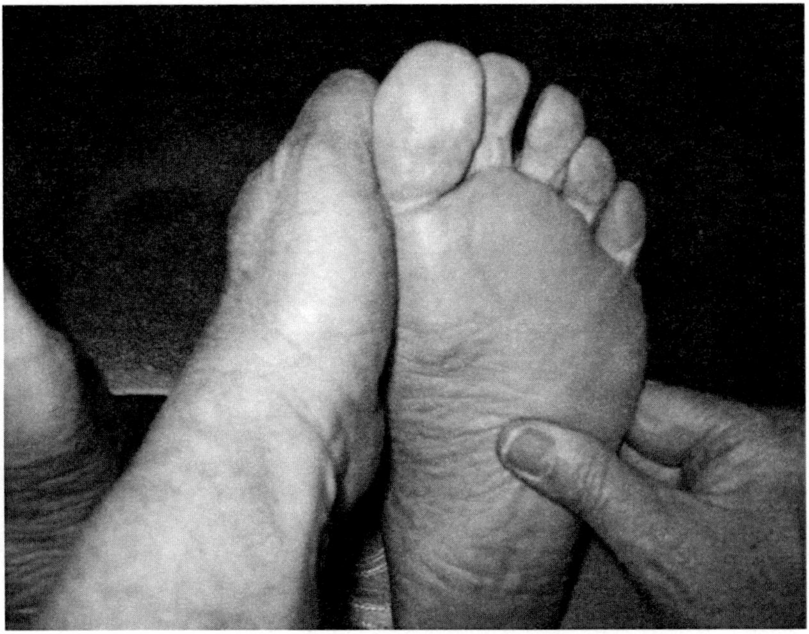

Stomach

Most of the reflex is found on the left foot and partly on the right. It is situated below the diaphragm and above the waist. Hold the toes gently taking care not to bend the large toe too far back when putting pressure on the thrusting forward tendon.

Holding with the left hand use the right hand to thumb walk a little below the diaphragm line from the inside of the foot to the centre of the foot

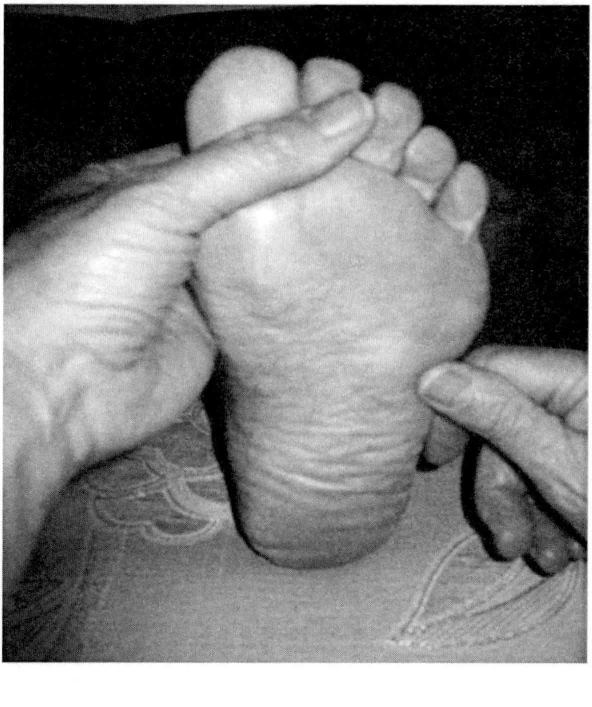

Pancreas

Remember most of this reflex is found on the left foot with only a small amount on the right foot. Use the right hand to steady the foot and thumb walk in the same way as for the stomach. This area consists of many organs.

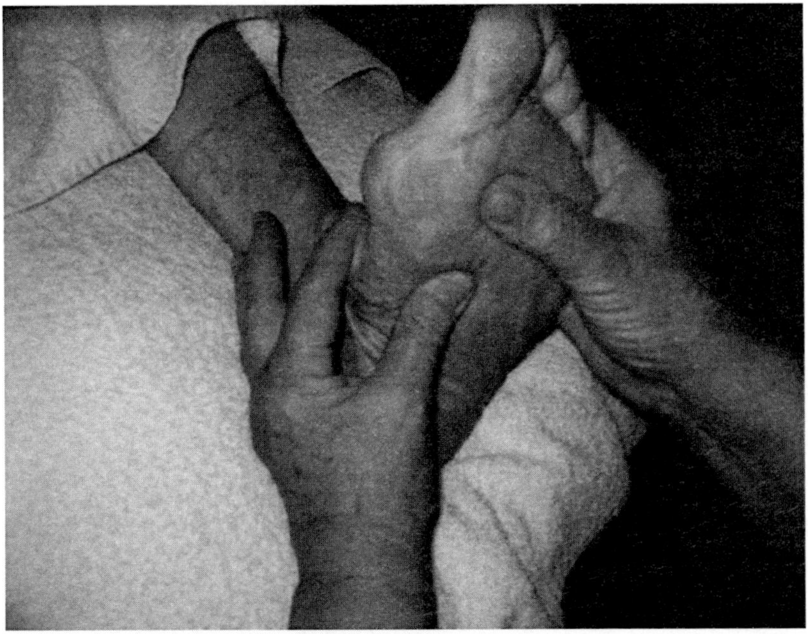

Liver

Previously discussed as one of the reflexes used in R.R.

A reflex, which students tend to forget, is on the right foot only.

Because it covers an area from waistline to diaphragm and from the inside to outside the foot a change of hands may be needed. Similarly to the stomach reflex, care must be taken when working across the tendon.

Reflexologists usually work the entire area when treating a condition and use the thumb to give gentle pressure

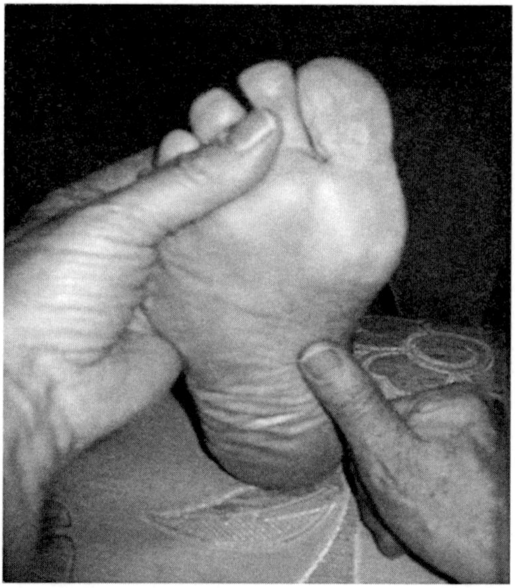

Gall Bladder

Another, right foot only, reflex. It is found in line with the fourth toe between the diaphragm line and the waistline. Hold the toes firmly but not tightly and use your working hand to press the pad of your thumb onto the gallbladder reflex. Press the thumb gently into the reflex while rotating the foot with the working hand.

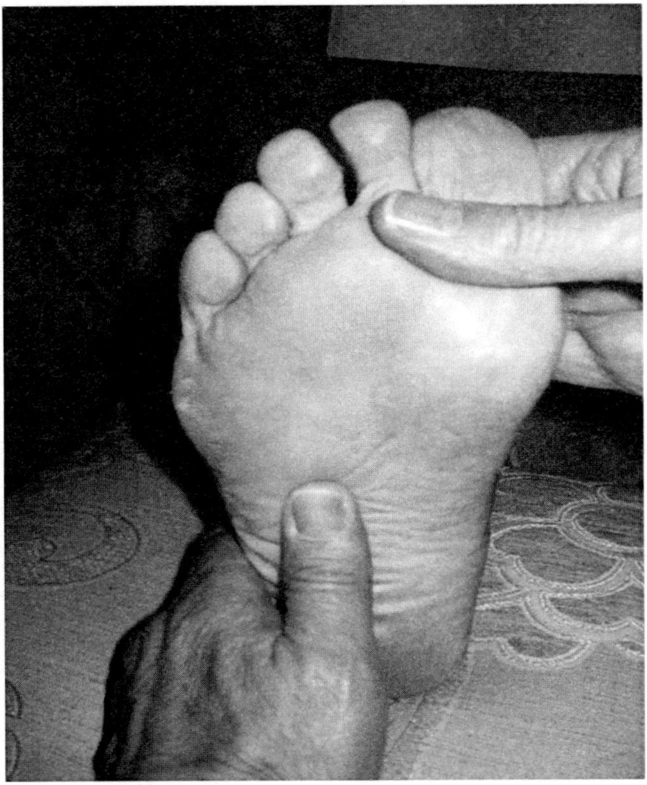

Adrenal gland

The adrenal glands can be worked best by first bending the toes back a little, until the tendon protrudes. The tendon runs from the big toe to the heel and the reflex point is found on the inside of the tendon, about halfway up the waistline to the diaphragm. Grip the top of the foot with the right hand, then thumb walk with the left hand on the reflex whilst rotating the foot into your thumb pressure.

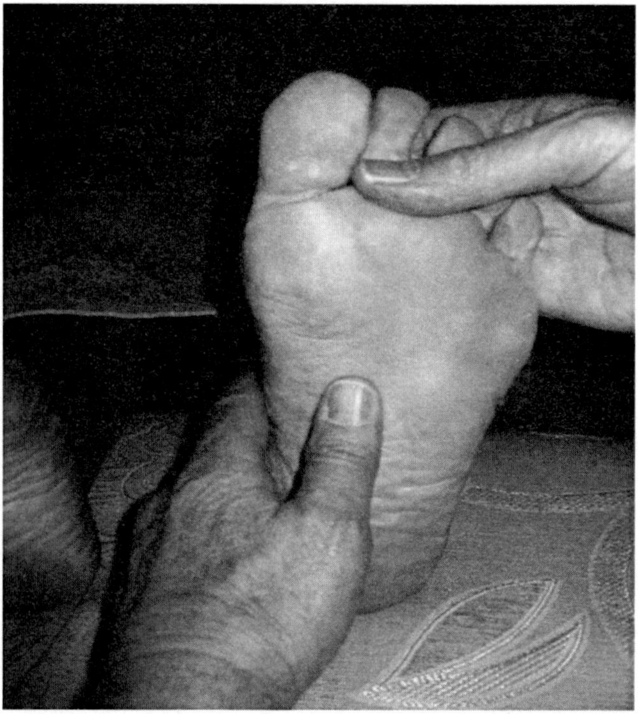

Kidney

Move the thumb down a little from the adrenal point to find the kidney reflex. Remember that part of the reflex is situated a little above the waistline and the other half, ureter tube and bladder just below the waistline. Use the tip of the thumb to give a slight pressure into the location, and give some circular motions very gently.

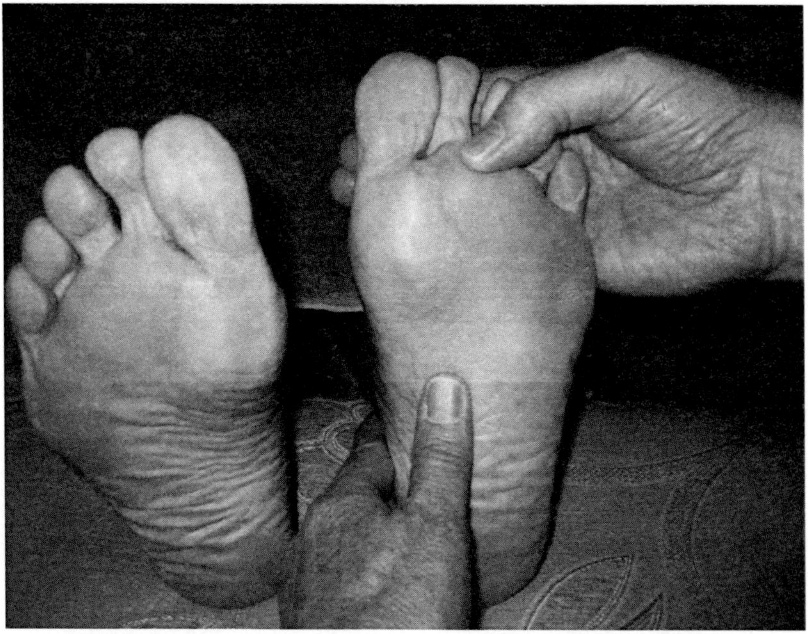

Ureter tube/bladder

The ureter reflex runs across the arch on the sole of the foot, from the kidney reflex to the bladder reflex. Caterpillar walk down the reflex onto the inside of the foot where the bladder reflex is located beneath the inner anklebone. Thumb walking or circular movements can be used on both areas

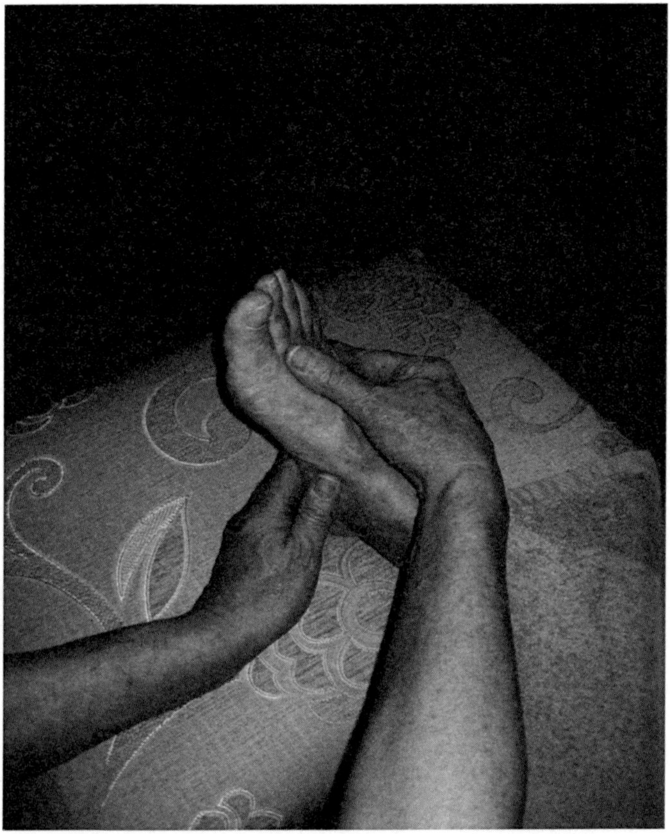

Intestines

The small intestine extends horizontally across the arch of the foot to below the fourth toe. Just above the pelvic line between the third and fourth toes a hollow spot can be found which is the ileocaecal valve reflex point. Press on the point, with the left thumb and use the circular movement over the area. Then caterpillar walk up the ascending colon, the reflex begins just below the ileocaecal valve reflex. The transverse colon extends across the entire foot. Remember the other half of the colon is found on the left foot where it turns downwards to become the descending colon reflex.

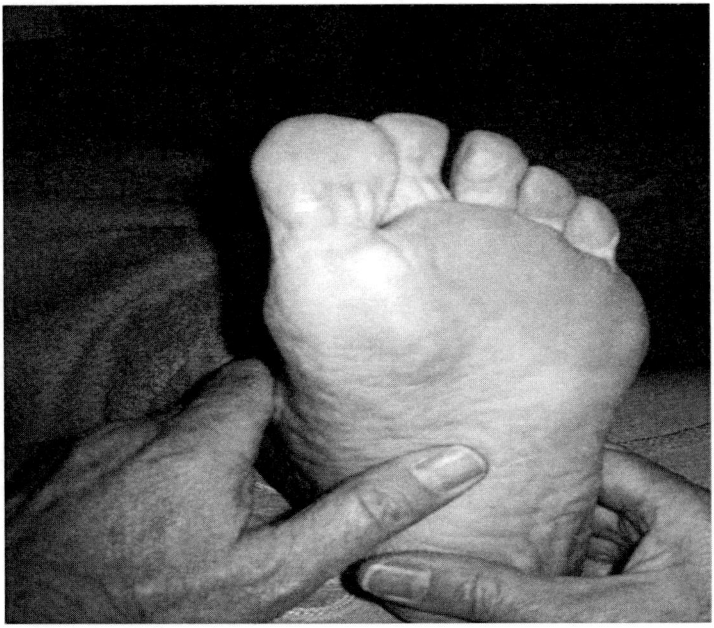

Arm and Shoulder

Use the holding hand to steady the foot and caterpillar walk vertically up the outer edge of the foot from the heel area to the little toe. Bearing in mind that the spine runs the length of the inside of the foot.

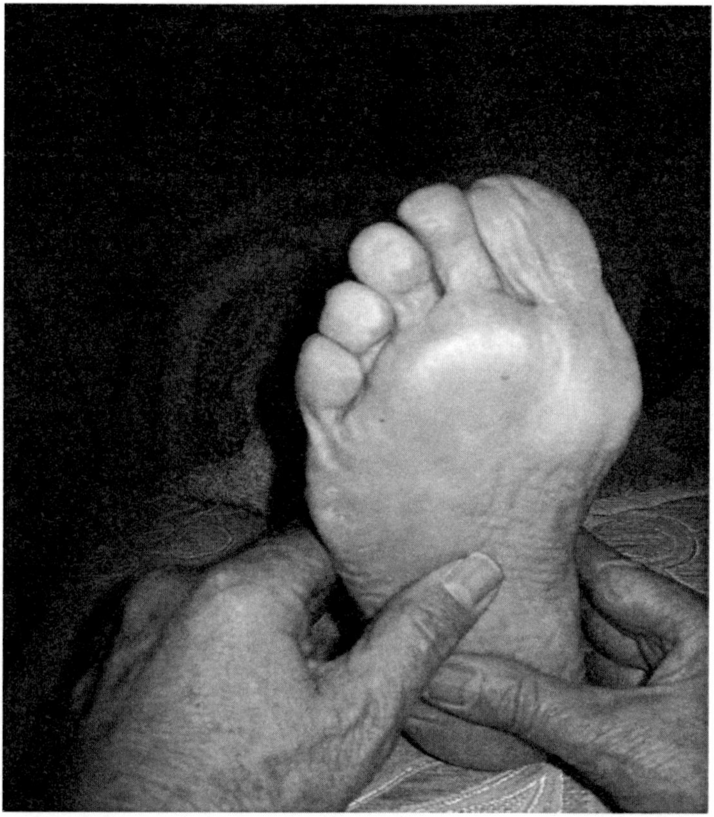

Spine

Hold the foot with the left hand and use the right hand to make gentle strokes down the inside of the foot from the base of the big toe down to the heel. To treat the entire reflex hold the foot under the heel and caterpillar walk down the inside of the foot starting from the toenail. Then thumb walk from the base of the heel up to the base of the toenail. To do this, place the holding hand around the top of the foot with the fingers holding the toes.

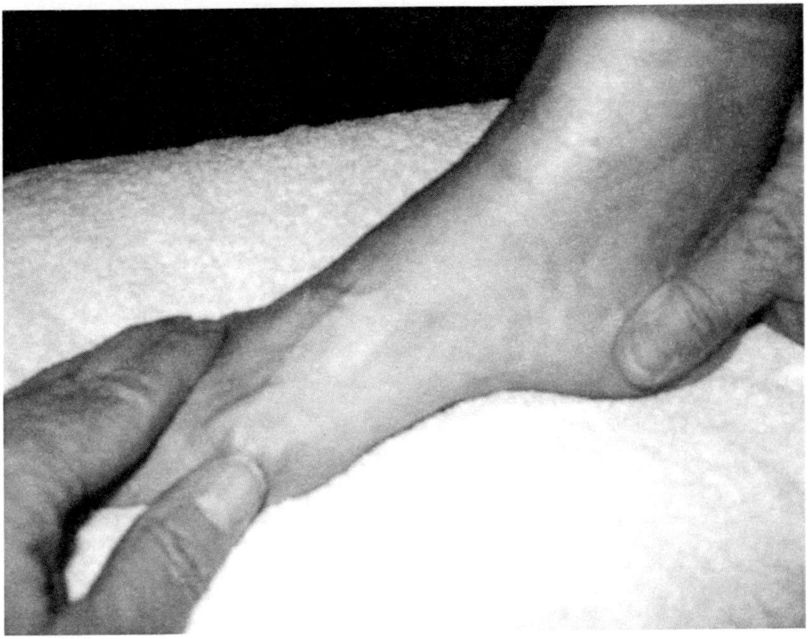

Hip

This area consists of a triangular indentation on the outside of the foot making up the leg and knee reflex and relating to the hip area. The finger walk technique is best on this reflex. It can be worked on from different directions.

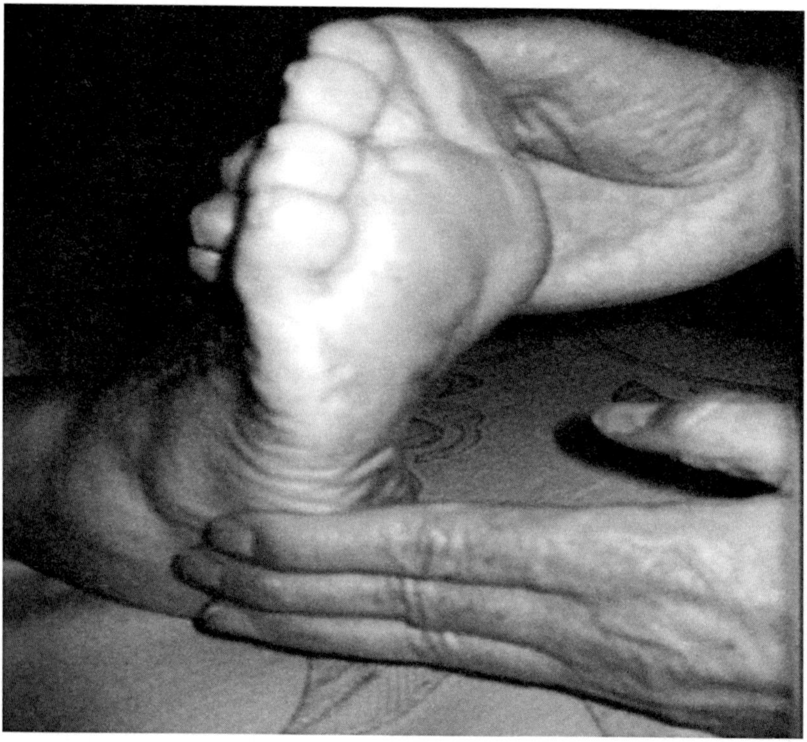

Sciatic nerve

In reflexology, this is an area not seen as a reflex but an actual nerve, which runs from the base of the heel up the leg and into the buttocks. It is a very sensitive area needing careful working. Use the left hand to hold and put the right thumb about six inches above the inner ankle bone. Thumb walk down the Achilles tendon area in the direction of the heel. You may find using the thumb difficult, if so finger walking is alright. I use the index finger to continue the walking up inside of leg behind the anklebone. Thumb walking is best along the sciatic nerve line on the bottom of the heel.

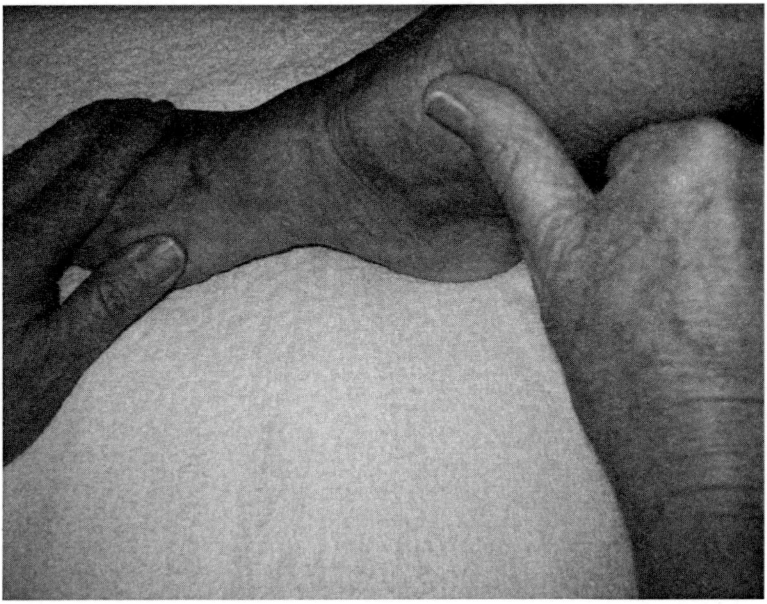

Ovaries and testicles

Located between the heel and anklebone on the outside of the foot. Imagine a diagonal from the base of the heel to the anklebone with the reflex point situated midway. The index finger is best for these points and should make small circular movements.

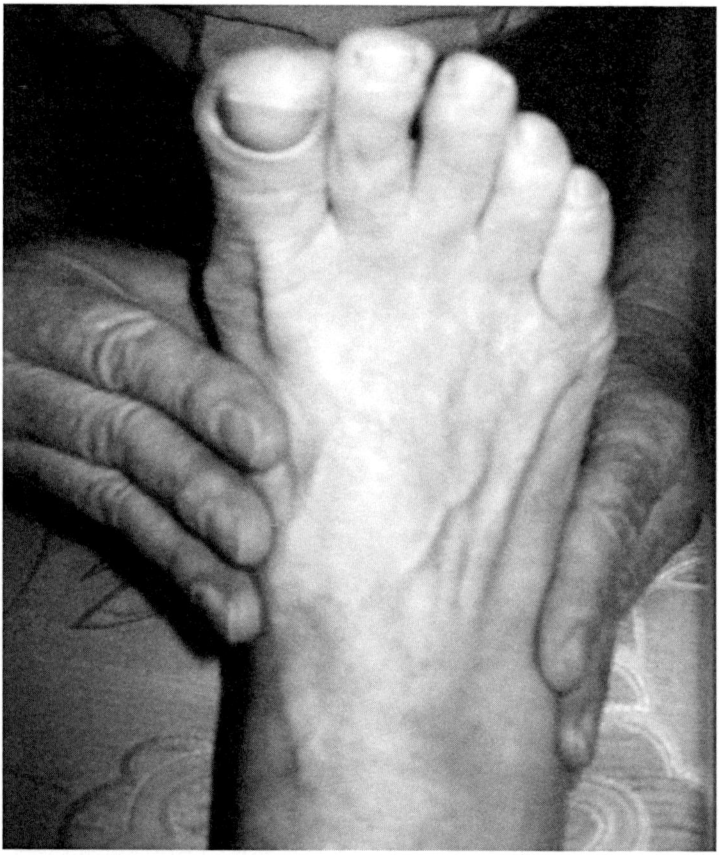

Lymphatic

These reflex points, found on top of the feet, between the first and second toes. It is the reflex area for the drainage of the lymphatics in the neck/chest region of the body. Hold the foot with the left hand to give support and use the right in carefully feeling the webbing between the toes, using the thumb and finger pressure.

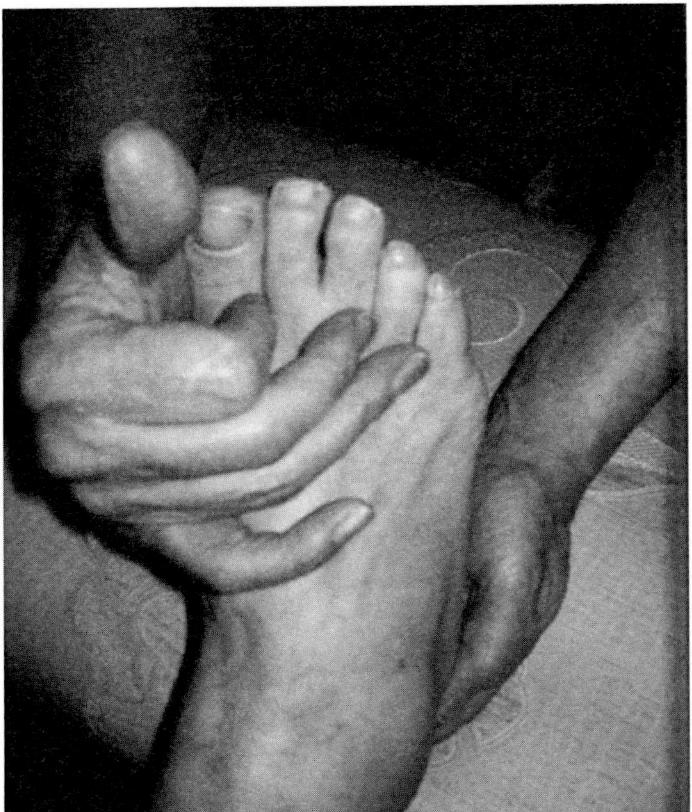

Uterus/prostate gland

Find the inner anklebone and put the index finger on, whilst placing your third finger on the tip of the heel. Then imagine a diagonal line between the two fingers. Midway on the line, from the base of the heel to the anklebone, is the uterus/prostate gland. Use a circular pressure on this area and finger walking is all right.

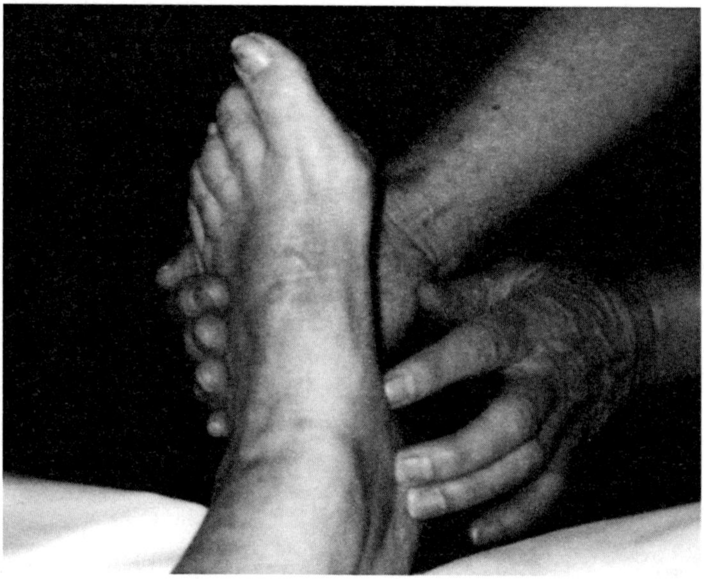

Groin/fallopian tube

The reflexes run across the top of the foot. They are sometimes worked on together with the reflexes of the ovaries and uterus. Use either thumb or finger walk from the inside of the ankle over the top of the foot to the outside of the ankle. It can be a tender area and should be gently worked on in both directions.

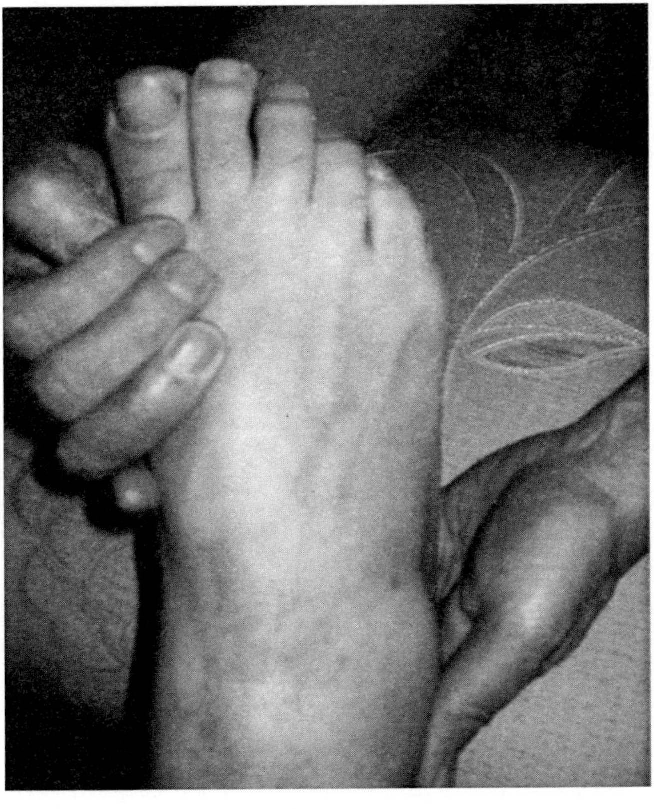

To finish each foot

Some reflexologists finish each foot by using the hook technique on the ankles. This is not only very relaxing, but can also clear toxins, possibly released during the session. Put both palms above the backsides of the heel and make smooth stroking movements, which moves the whole foot backwards, and forwards. It is necessary to keep the palms firmly in place around the anklebones. The technique needs thorough practise to get the right effect.

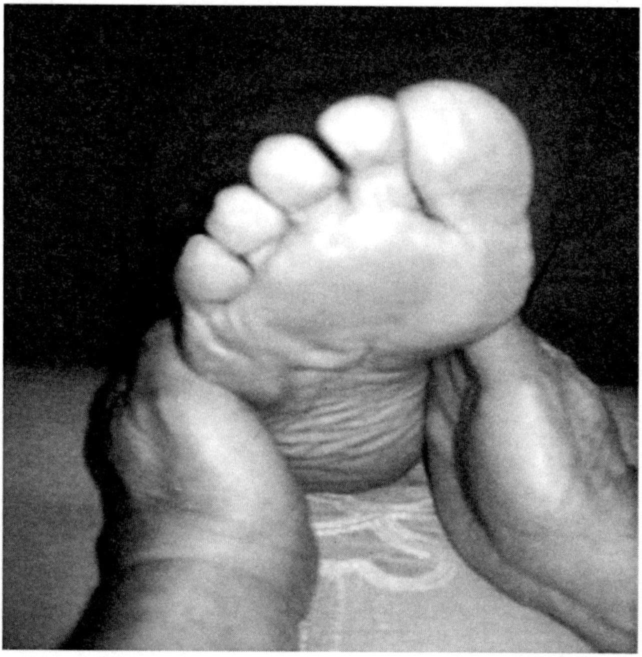

Foot Notes from case files

A young man came to me for reflexology treatment. His problem was moods of depression, which left him unable to relax. I gave him a full reflexology session and then suggested the R.R. technique. He asked for some notes explaining the exercises. After showing him how to carry out the procedure for homework, he decided to try two ten minute sessions a week for a trial. He received a full reflexology treatment from me once a week and carried out his own R.R. sessions twice a week.

After six weeks, he reported that he felt more lively and motivated to "drag himself out of his fits of depression".

A young woman, who seemed to be very anxious, came to me for reflexology because she was suffering from insomnia. I suggested she used the R.R. therapy a few times a week. After three weeks, she informed me that she felt much more relaxed and was sleeping very well. More than that, she was extremely pleased to find patches of eczema were less itchy and had improved immensely.

A student remarked to me that the sessions gave him a calmness he had not experienced before. Moreover, he thought his ability to concentrate was much better since he began having reflexology and R.R. treatment combined. He went on to say that, since the sessions, he was much better on letting go of tension and could relax more easily than previously

Due to what he called, "a nervous condition" a businessman explained how he had used R.R. to assist him in relaxing. He made time for three periods a week, consisting of thirty minutes before lunch. First, he locked his office door so there could be no disturbance. After removing his shoes and socks, he then gently stroked the reflexes whilst meditating on a relaxing scene from his memory.

He was positive that these periods of calm enabled him to “combat the strain of his work and keep his energy balanced".

A mother of five children explained to me how the sessions were benefiting her family. After learning how to use the reflexes to relax herself she taught it to her family. Particular times each week were used for giving each other a relaxing treatment under her supervision.

Through using R.R. as a family therapy she believed that help was given to her family on many levels; "mental, physical, spiritual and emotional"

It appeared to her that the family had become more aware of themselves in being able to help each other. There was a deeper interaction in understanding their problems and the family as a whole.

A male recipient first came to me for a full reflexology treatment because he was experiencing extreme fatigue. I took down his medical history and he assured me that he was not suffering from any medical condition. His past health history had been good, although he had been going through a very emotional time, which had left him in a state of excessive anxiety.

His doctor could not find any physical symptoms accounting for his tiredness and lack of energy. I suspected that he was very stressed out. After giving the feet a relaxing general treatment, I gave him some exercises for homework.

He received one full reflexology session a week and gave himself three twenty-minute R.R. treatments during the course of a week. He responded by explaining to me that after six weeks of the course he felt "refreshed and full of energy". The time he allowed for treatment had, in his words, "helped him to get problems into perspective".

A forty-year-old female claimed the therapy had helped her to change her lifestyle for the better. She was certain this had come about because she felt more relaxed and full of energy. As a result giving up smoking had been easy along with healthier eating habits.

The recipient believed she had gained a much more positive mental attitude to improving her health. Furthermore, as she developed skill, the therapy helped her circulation problem.

An elderly woman gained more than one benefit from treatment. During the first session I found her feet were tense and the toes lacked flexibility. I suggested she tried some specific exercises to loosen her feet as well as using the reflexes.

A few months later, after she had become proficient in using the exercises, she was delighted to find there was less discomfort in her feet, the circulation had improved and she felt more relaxed.

When stiffness and tension are removed in the feet, the results can be quite remarkable. It is not uncommon for headaches to be the result of badly functioning feet. Many of the claims made for the healing power of reflexology, is due in my opinion, to little more than its ability to help feet lose their stiffness and tension.

Hand Exercises for the Reflex-Relaxologist

These exercises will relax the hands and help to keep the thumb and finger joints, strong, supple and flexible. In addition, if you keep a quiet mind and uninterrupted concentration you can find the exercises very relaxing.

Begin by loosely shaking the hands from the wrists downwards. Then rub both hands together to improve the circulation. Hold the hands out in front of you and separate the fingers. Try to make circles with the fingers without moving the wrists. Next bring the fingers together in a firm press that will help to tone and strengthen them.

You are now prepared to carry out the fingers and thumb exercises. Begin by holding the thumb of one hand with the thumb and index finger of the working hand and gently massage from the base to the top. Keep the hand stationary and move the thumb in circular movements with the thumb and forefinger of the working hand.

Finish off with a pettrisage movement over the palm of each hand. In massage terms pettrisage is described as a kneading movement similar to kneading dough, and used to relieve tension and stiffness in the muscles. Use your thumb to make a creeping pettrisage massage over each palm in turn which will improve the circulation all over your hand.

When you are doing these exercises, view it as time spent preparing your tools (hands) for working effectively.

Chapter Six

Treating a Partner

The main skill needed to give or receive R.R. from a partner is the ability to create a relaxing atmosphere. To do this we have to be "user-friendly" and initiate a healing process. There must be no embarrassment or tension involved. It should be a time for positive emotions of, giving or receiving healing, whether he/she is your wife, husband, daughter, son, or friend. Do not worry about getting the technique right when you first begin. It is more important to get a reassuring feedback that neither of you are experiencing any discomfort.

Start the treatment off by analysing each other's feet. Remember the same consideration must be given, to whether treatment is appropriate in the case of any illness or injury, you or your partner may have. Observe any ingrowing toenail, bunion, or corns, because these problems will interfere with the therapy. If any problem areas are found on the feet there is a possibility that they could effect the corresponding part of the body. It is important that any irritations on the feet be addressed before R.R. takes place. When you are both satisfied that you have no foot problems, which could give a negative effect on the body, you can start using the method on each other.

The whole purpose of the therapy is to give relaxation to each other therefore do not omit the special foot massage discussed earlier. The massage is just as important as the reflex areas are, so you must practice it very carefully before working on the selected reflexes. You can warm up the feet by first massaging the sole of each foot in turn. Best carried out by using small rotary movements with the thumbs. Cover the whole area of the foot. If you do this on your own feet and cannot find a comfortable way to have, the sole positioned for thumb walking, try using your fingertips underneath the foot. Do not use your knuckles because the hard pressure could damage the tendon, felt in the arch of the foot, particularly when you bend the big toe back. Always be very careful not to force the toes back too far with the holding hand causing the tendon to jut out and feel taut.

After you have practiced and studied the exercises in this book, you should feel competent enough to guide your partner into giving you a feeling of total relaxation from the therapy. Then you can return the favour to your partner by giving them a well-practiced session of relaxation, bearing in mind that the professional reflexologist always takes a medical history before giving a first treatment. So you do need to be sure that treatment is not inappropriate to any condition your partner is suffering from.

When giving treatment, look occasionally at your partner's face, in order to notice any sign of grimace, or discomfort. If there is find out why? As you practice, you will become aware that different parts of the foot are more sensitive than other parts. Therefore, it will be necessary to change the amount of pressure used. See the technique as giving healing and not in the sense of massaging a pair of feet. Take care not to dig in your nails, or to press too hard, otherwise you may be causing pain and discomfort instead of relaxation.

Some reflexologists recommend the use of foot rollers and other instruments for home use. My advice is that no instruments, other than the fingers and thumbs should be used for R.R. The hands are the only tools that can give precise pressure and regulate the correct amount needed. You cannot detect with sensitivity, or feel acid crystal deposits with some hard instrument; such skill comes gradually after much practice.

Use the sessions to become aware of your whole self. It can help you to focus on your lifestyle and think about how you are treating your body. In a way you are monitoring your own stress by becoming more aware of your tensions and how they can be gradually eased by the workouts.

The 3Rs for Children

Children today are probably under as much pressure and stress as their parents (in some cases more). In my experience as a teacher, I have seen the harmful effects anxiety can have on a child. It can be devastating to their intellectual achievement and detrimental to social and personal development. In some cases, every area of their school life altered for the worse. Today, in education, emphasis is placed upon academic achievement and only platitudes are made to consider children's anxieties.

Prolonged stress in a child may lead to all kinds of complications. Many behavioural problems, at school or in the home, can be due to stress. Undue pressure on children can trigger off physical reactions, such as, stomach pain, skin rashes,. even difficulties with sleeping and breathing problems. The common outcome, evident to teachers in particular, is the profound effect harmful stress as on a child's learning ability. Concentration is low and some children become withdrawn and have tearful spells.

R.R. is a constructive way in which parents can play a role in dealing with helping children cope with stress. Every good mother or father is conscious of a teaching and healing awareness towards their children. By studying the system outlined in this book, they can acquire an ideal skill to benefit everyone in the home. With a little practice, they will find it possible to build up an invaluable talent to give more understanding and support within the family setting.

Students participating in workshops have surprised me by telling me of the many ways they have helped members of their family by combining the technique with a counselling session. Because they have experienced what the therapy can achieve they are able to explain the difference between feeling tense and relaxed after treatment. More than this, it becomes their own individual method of using a session to discuss emotional difficulties.

It becomes a positive tool for a caring parent to help their family on a physical and psychological level. In many cases an understanding and closer relationship is formed. What better way than during this relaxing period is a parent able to give counselling time to a listening child? Opportunity arises to renew what may be a lost bonding process. As one parent put it, "I have gained a skill which not only helps me to relax but also helps me to communicate better with my family". It then becomes a two way process and the parent benefits as much as the child.

Parents become a therapist and contribute to the healing process. By so doing, they are giving support and comfort, which in turn can release their own frustrations of feeling helpless. Instead of relying only on experts, they can use their own healing skills inherent in everyone. They are not acting as a professional but identifying a problem that may need professional help.

When a parent is confident to act as a therapist in this way, they have told me how it seems to build up trust in a child. Then when they become aware of the parents hands in contact with his/her feet an ideal healing state takes place. Hyperactive children are calmed down and lethargic ones receive energy and stimulation. Without doubt, if used properly, it is a time when relaxation can take over from fears and anxiety.

Parents, over time, are able to perfect a health care skill. A complementary technique to aid orthodox medical care. It not only helps the child to cope with illness, but also assists in their recuperation afterwards.

It was during my years as the head teacher of a special school I was privileged to work with parents interested in the principles of reflexology. They believed, as I did, that it could be a relaxing aid to help their children. It was mainly from these experiences that the R.R. therapy began. Thanks to the co-operation of those parents, I was able to pursue research into its use for relaxing body and mind. The following gives suggestions for using the treatment in a family setting.

Using the Technique as Counselling Therapy Within the Family

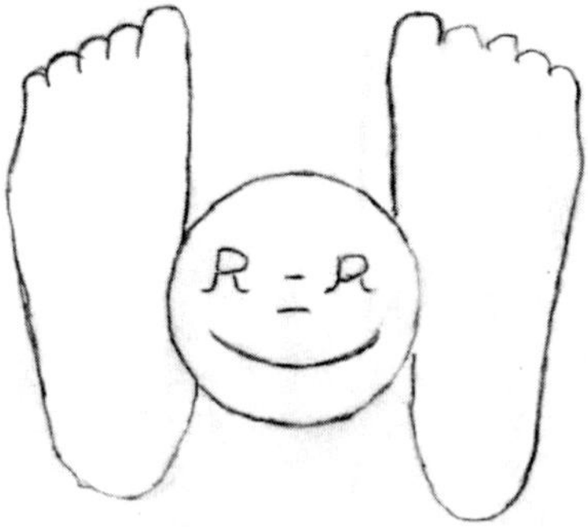

A relaxed body will improve a child physically, mentally, and emotionally. He/she will be able to think more clearly. When a parent becomes a R.R. therapist, they have the means, readily available, to induce a favourable condition for the release of subconscious anxiety in children. As a parent, you can combine the therapy with the following procedure.

If possible, the treatment should take place in the surroundings of the child's home. Choose a quiet room where you will not be disturbed or interrupted. It needs to be a warm room because when socks are taken off feet may become cold. Just before bedtime is ideal for the session. They will not have had a large meal and the treatment will encourage restful sleep. For younger children you can motivate their interest and co-operation by showing them the R.R. Logo picture of the happy looking face. This pairing of an image with the session can promote a pleasant frame of mind. More than this, it can also help a childs ability to relax by associating relaxation with the smiling logo. Parents have told me how they have achieved amazing results with children by using the simple logo visual technique. It enabled them to create a relaxation-inducing image by which a child is able to identify with a relaxed mental and physical state.

Always view the session spent with children, however long you make it, as a time for counselling. It is a period, to make an opportunity, for discussion about their lifestyle and consequently anxieties. For instance, how are they getting on at school? Have they any problems with their peers or teachers?

It can also be a very appropriate time for a child to tell you about any aches or pains he/she may have. Obviously, foot care can be discussed. The necessity to cut nails and the importance of keeping feet clean. Are there any marks or deformities apparent on the feet? Consequently, a parent becomes health educator and counsellor, as well as helping the child to open up and talk about problems. If for no other reason than this, you are perfecting a worthwhile skill for any parent to have.

A Comfortable Position

As you begin the therapy, it is important to check posture. Otherwise the recipient may not gain the full benefit of treatment. Your body must be in a position, which does not cause discomfort to yourself. Also, make sure the recipient's body is supported in a way that will not interfere with their relaxation.

In the case of a child sitting or lying in an awkward position, he/she is more likely to feel pain rather than be in a relaxed state. In a tensed up unnatural form they will be more inclined to resist the therapy than to participate. Any imbalanced posture will result in fatigue. For these reasons, workshops in teaching the method give attention to the correct body position.

Facilitate Relaxation

In treating children's feet, proceed with the same caution previously mentioned in working with adults. In particular, you must be very patient in gaining the right amount of light pressure and be fully aware of not spending too long on one area.

Try using a little talcum powder on the feet, which will help you find the specific points without slipping off. Begin by holding the foot in both hands and gently using the thumbs to stroke upwards over the arch and ball to the top of the toes. This will help to tone up the circulation and prepare the feet for treatment.

Don't forget to treat both feet in the same way to give a balanced effect.

Then use your thumbs to give single point pressure to the solar plexus to calm the nervous system. Use your thumb and fingers and gently pull out each toe as though you were trying to straighten them. By starting out with these exercises, you will have begun to facilitate relaxation in your child. Then you can carry out the complete system.

A Successful Session

Remember to keep the atmosphere friendly and do not show any irritation from the start to finish of the session. Choose a time convenient to both of you. It would be foolish to imagine a profitable outcome taking place if your child wanted to watch a favourite TV programme. Keep the therapy unhurried so that you can give it all your attention. Give encouragement if they want to discuss any problems or anxieties.

Use the opportunity to teach your child to cope with stress from an early age. If nothing else, you are able to listen and perhaps sooth away tensions. Until gradually you are able to prove during the session that relaxation is the body's natural antidote to anxiety. At the same time you are becoming more skilled in opening up a new source of communication within the family.

Chapter Seven

A Foot in the Hand Instead of the Grave

A skill for the Senior Citizen

R.R. can enhance the quality of life for senior citizens on many different levels. Its study during the senior years can add to the maturing wisdom that develops with advancing time. A new achievement made, which gives benefit to themselves and others.

This is without minimizing or over-simplifying the realities of the aging process. There can be extremely high stress levels to contend with, as one gets older. Quite often age brings many unforeseen changes in circumstances. The senior citizen in today's world has to come to terms with a rapidly changing way of life, which they may find difficult to understand. Many are living on their own after bereavement and in need of special care and counselling. Loneliness and isolation are common stress-related problems for many elderly people.

Such situations can mean very little opportunity for the older person to communicate his/her fears and anxiety. In many cases, they have no one who they can confide in. Gradually their self-esteem becomes low as they give way to an outlook of worthlessness.

I have seen R.R. put back quality into the lives of people living with the problems mentioned. They used an opportunity which gave them therapy and a skill to practice. Instead of feeling left out they discovered the joy of making oneself available to help others be it sons, daughters, grandchildren, or family friends. It becomes a means to many ends. Not only are they contributing to life in a healing sense but also they can use the skill to bring young and old together with remarkable results. It can be a medium to break down the generation gap. Some elderly people have remarked that since they have practised the skills with their grandchildren, a closer bond has developed.

The older person is ideally suited to the study and practice of R.R. In fact even more than the younger person. They have a great potential which is very often untapped. It is the accumulated knowledge and experience of life, which through the study of this therapy can be nourished and developed. They are able to bring to the subject of relaxation a wisdom that cannot be gleaned from textbooks. It has been gained from real life experience that teaches the art of accepting the bitter with the sweet.

I undertook the following survey to find out what benefits the elderly student had in learning how to use R.R. The results appeared to be mainly on four levels; physical, mental, social, and in their relationships.

Physically they felt less stressed and their circulation improved which is important in old age. They also believed that practising relaxation gave them a sense of being physically active. They thought the mental effort needed to gain the simple skills for giving treatment was attainable and enjoyable. The study enabled them to bring their own experience to the therapy. It is a study which encourages creativity. Some of them realised expertise, gained dearly, in their professional life could be of immense value. They were able to add counselling skills to that of R.R. relaxation.

It gave them the opportunity to be more socially active because they were mixing with a like minded group of people interested in a form of healing. A consequence of retirement is a decreasing interaction with society. Such a state can leave the individual with a sense of uselessness. They now, not only had a worthwhile aim in life, but also, the cheerful, friendly chatter that can be sorely missed upon retirement from daily work.

New relationships were developed in the workshops which gave them an opportunity to communicate. They were able to use the treatment at the same time as talking through problems with trusted relatives or friends. Such communication, in itself, is particularly therapeutic for taking the stress out of a situation. Explaining, or demonstrating, the technique became a purposeful way of gaining new relations with others.

Special Care Needed

It is important that, as well as the normal cautions needed, further safety regards be considered for senior citizens. The older person's joints may be stiff and toes bent. Therefore, a much lighter and gentle touch is used.

Small blood vessels in the feet are prone to break as we age and care must be taken regarding the amount of pressure put on such areas. Do not twist your joints or damage other parts of your body by trying to stretch out your legs. Find any comfortable position without unduly stretching any stiff joints into contortions. The same applies if you are giving treatment to others. It is unnecessary and harmful to use force.

When carried out with care R.R. can give relief from stress and anxiety states common to older people. I look forward to the time when it will be available on the National Health Service.

Use the Technique to Aid Foot Care

A further benefit comes from studying the pressure points on feet. It will gradually increase awareness and understanding of how healthy feet influence our physical and mental well-being. Unhealthy feet cause the reverse effect and in some cases will cause pain in other areas of the body.

Most people seem to pay little attention to foot care until some problem arises. It is very rare in my work as a reflexologist to find an adult with perfect feet. There is usually some defect that could have been avoided. Although a reflexologist can point out foot defects they can only be treated by a qualified chiropodist.

The human foot consists of 26 bones forming a series of arches supported by ligaments, muscles and tendons. Although it is a strong structure, it is also a delicate, complex form easily damaged. At the age of about eighteen, the bones are fully set. Before this period, it is important that children's future foot health is considered, although adults feet can still be damaged usually by ill-fitting shoes.

R.R. encourages and educates individuals into looking after the feet, by enhancing observation and therapeutic touch. The simple act of laying hands on the feet can give greater relaxation than laying them on other parts of the body, and gradually a person becomes more attuned to what their feet can tell them. For instance if they were working on a pressure point on one of the toes they would soon become aware of any ingrowing toenail from the amount of pain received. Ingrown toenails are quite a common sight in my work and the sufferer is advised to see a chiropodist before I give any reflexology treatment. The cause is usually a splinter of nail entering the side of the toe and sticking into the flesh. Sometimes the side of the nail is removed under local anaesthesia. Alternatively, in severe cases the podiatrist recommends that the whole nail be removed. So the prevention of ingrowing toenail's should be taken seriously.

It is especially in the toes where many foot disorders occur. They become misshapen, bent, and cause incorrect bone alignment to form. Once a toe becomes out of shape it is very difficult to straighten it gain. Consequently, it is the cause of other deformities arising. Once toes are out of shape, the shock-absorbing effect of the forefoot throws it out of balance. If proper care is taken in childhood defects can be avoided.

R.R. is a very positive way for a parent to identify foot problems and monitor treatment which can be given by a qualified chiropodist. Parents can also use the session as a hygiene remedial function. Children will be able to experience that washing the feet sometimes is not just a matter of cleanliness but also a remedial function if the pre-technique system for treatment, explained earlier, is used. Looked at in this way, bathing the feet becomes not merely a matter of cleanliness, but will help to soothe tired and strained feet.

When foot health is not maintained consequences can be very drastic in later life, In fact foot problems among the elderly, in some cases, have been recorded as causing loss of mobility, resulting in a need for residential care.

A partner, friend, or member of the family whilst giving a therapy session to an elderly person is able to monitor and advise them about the condition of their feet which may prevent foot troubles later in life.

If an elderly persons, feet give too much pain to walk on they become less active at a time when mobility is a priority. In many cases they show a loss of general interest and become homebound. A lack of exercise and interest in life leads to many ills, which may be avoided with a little foot care.

When you become more skilled in using the therapy detailed in this book you will be able to detect tension and stress through feeling the texture of the skin. It is possible, with experience, to become aware of degenerative changes to the skin. In old age, it becomes thin and dry. Also because of partial wasting of fatty tissue, underlying parts receive greater pressure and irritation, particularly on the weight-bearing region of the feet. Your hands can feel these lesions. It is important that such lesions receive professional expertise before the tissues break down and perhaps ulcerate.

Therefore, you are able to use your skills not only for giving yourself and others relaxation, but also as an excellent aid to checking foot problems. Of course, you should never attempt to treat unhealthy conditions that need the help of specialists.

A Partnership

When you give yourself R.R. you are working in partnership with reflexology. Furthermore, it can be complementary to orthodox medicine. It should not be seen as alternative to medical treatment. View it as a gentle therapy, used to suit an individual's response to stress.

The method does not make any unrealistic quasi-scientific claims, or use any poorly defined concepts. Many therapies are far too unclear in their use of terminology. If complementary therapy is to become totally accepted by orthodox medicine, it must be well evaluated and attempt, other than anecdotal, to quantify the basis for its use. In orthodox medicine, new technology is making remarkable advances to the extension of life. Reflex-relaxology contributes by giving more quality to life.

Despite advances in treating illness, both medical and natural healers must accept that, as yet, neither medical nor natural healers, have found any one miracle to cure illness.

It is now understood many illnesses are the result of stress. The treatment outlined in this book consists in the use of a simple technique that has its basis in relaxation therapy. It is a self-help skill designed to relieve stress and by so doing forms a partnership with health care, within a realistic view of its limitations.

Chapter Eight

Other Therapies Relevant to Stress related disorders

It should be noted that most of these therapies are not subjected to the clinical tests that doctors carry out on treatments that are orthodox. Nor is there any scientific foundation behind most of them. Therefore, use caution, in judging whether they can help you. I have not attempted to judge or assess the value of the therapies. I believe it is probably best to view them as aids to healing, rather than cures.

Homeopathy

I include this one because it is concerned with preventing illness as well as treatment. It is a system of medicine which believes that "like cures like". It was formulated by a German physician, called Dr. Samuel Hahnemann (1755-1843). He experimented with the medical drugs in use at the time, and found that to dilute the strength of a drug by shaking it up in water did not weaken it but increased its effect. Consequently, he called his dilution a "succussion" or "potentising" the drug. Homeopathic remedies use extremely small doses of the original substances, which gives the reason for many doctors to doubt its success for curing illness. In recent years controlled tests have been undertaken which have proved effective in treating some diseases.

In many cases, it is possible to use both conventional medicine and homeopathic remedies that can complement each other. Many chiropodists are now using homoeopathic remedies in their practice: for example, homoeopathic arnica can be used with normal treatment, for pain in the big toe, sometimes caused by gout, or homoeopathic ledum is used if the toe becomes swollen from the condition. Arundo is prescribed for offensive sweaty feet. When both soles of the feet and the hands burn, homoeopathic sulphur is suggested.

Homeopathy views the individual as being unique and treats the whole person. The remedies are selected not only on symptoms of an illness but also on the person's disposition and appearance.

Acupuncture

The word acupuncture means, "needle piercing". It is a traditional Chinese medical treatment dating back to 2697 B.C. Recent use suggests it might control pain and possibly treat stress-related disorders. Practitioners have to reach a high level of skill in being able to place very fine needles into the skin without causing pain. Electro or laser treatment is sometimes used, instead of needles.

The theory is that the body has an invisible energy flow (chi) that runs throughout the body along channels named meridians. The concept is that the channels are linked to a persons internal organs. If the energy flow becomes blocked then illness will take place.

It is important to let an acupuncturist know if you have a cardiac pacemaker or any cosmetic implant. Always be careful to give the practitioner information regarding any pre-existing conditions you may have. The therapist must be aware if you are, or could be, pregnant. He must also know the names of any medicines you are taking.

Acupressure

Acupressure is similar to acupuncture, but without the use of needles. It originates from China and uses a system of finger pressures to press on the meridian points of the body (the special channels of magnetic energy)

The main concept for this therapy is a belief that when gentle finger pressure is placed upon the channels the energy flow is stimulated and the release of endorphins (the body's painkillers) takes place.

Like acupuncture, it believes in treating the individual as a whole. Both physical and mental health is considered. As in acupuncture, it is believed when the energy flow is corrected, body and mind will gain the right state of balance and as a result healing can take place.

Too much pressure on the acupoints will produce pain and can be dangerous when used on the points at the base of the skull.

Shiatsu

I include this summary of shiatsu because of its strong reliance on "touch information" between practitioner and recipient. The physical technique is combined with an awareness of psychological and spiritual implications. A shiatsu practitioner believes that touch can improve physical well-being.

This therapy is also similar to acupuncture and acupressure. The word means "finger pressure". It is a Japanese healing system developed from 4000 years of Oriental medicine. No needles are used, and works with the idea that the practitioner and recipient use the healing ability of both to balance the life force known as Qi (pronounced 'chi' in China, 'ki' in Japan).

The system of treatment relies on the individual being responsible for his or her own health. It also states the theory that situated in the foot are nerve endings from all over the body and consequently body illness is mirrored in the foot. Foot massage is quite often used by the. Practitioner and is sometimes used to energise tired feet. The therapist using the ball of the thumb, not the tip, and exerting pressure for five to seven seconds carries this out.

There is a lot of confusion regarding its safety as a self-help technique so it is best to take treatment from a qualified practitioner.

Biofeedback

This is a method of monitoring personal stress levels and by so doing achieving relaxation. It is a scientific technique formulated in the 1960s, for measuring physical responses to stress. The biofeedback machine does not alter or affect the body in any way. It merely enables the individual to see for him or herself how stress can change their mental and physical condition.

The information gained from the machine is used by a practitioner to teach the individual how to control and assess certain bodily responses and by so doing could be able to avoid conditions such as high blood pressure. It is now recognised that a person can, with training, become aware of, and change muscular tension, blood pressure, and skin temperature, which once were thought to be involuntary responses.

Treatment is usually undertaken by the recipient sitting in front of the biofeedback machine. Electrode sensors (wires) on the machine will be connected to him or her and relaxation techniques will be used by the practitioner to relax the person. They will then be asked to reduce their tension or slow down their heart rate. During this time the machine is measuring heart rate, muscle rate, muscle tension, blood flow, and so on, giving feedback via beeps, pictures, or graphic lines.

It is now a common treatment for many stress related disorders, and used by qualified practitioners, can augment other therapies dealing with stress control.

Bach Flower Remedies

Bach flower remedies are often used in conjunction with reflexology. The remedies were developed by Dr Edward Bach (1880-1936), an English Doctor who started his career as a pathologist bacteriologist. He at first experimented with homeopathy but later believed that different diseases seemed to be linked to the various temperaments of his patients. He classified their character types into twelve archetypes although later on he added 26 more new remedies to the original. The remedies were given for emotional states such as fear or loneliness. Plants were put together which he believed would make the negative emotional states become positive. In this way it was thought that the remedies helped to relieve a persons physical symptoms associated with the emotional state.

There is not much published scientific work on the Bach flower remedies and although they use the 'essences' of flowers and trees, they are more homeopathic than herbal in the way they are said to work. Practitioners at first are not basically concerned about the patients physical condition but more with their emotional state. He/she helps the patient to face inner feelings of envy, jealousy, guilt, or even hatred, in order to find which remedy may meet their condition. Once they have been treated for the type of person they are, then the practitioner looks for improvement in any physical problem.

The remedies are usually taken orally, or used as a lotion compress, hot fermentation, or added to a bath. Despite the fact that no one has explained scientifically how the remedies work, they are used throughout the world.

Aromatherapy

Aromatherapy is gaining in popularity as a complimentary therapy. It claims to have been practised in the ancient world, like reflexology notably by the Egyptians. A chemist named

Rene'-Maurice Gattefosse revived the therapy in the 1920s. After accidentally burning his hand, he put it into some lavender oil and became aware how quickly the pain ceased and the skin healed, without blistering.

Aromatherapy uses oils to treat the body. The concentrated oils are known as 'essential oils' extracted from plants, leaves, seeds, and flowers, reputed to have healing properties. Research has confirmed that essential oils massaged into the skin will move into the bloodstream and the lymphatic system within four hours. They are believed to relax, tone, and improve mobility in the body and certain oil smells are thought to help people suffering from anxiety or depression. The oils are not just used for massage, they are sometimes used as steam inhalation.

When used in massage they can generally provide a very relaxing effect and many aromatherapists combine the massage with a reflexology treatment.

The oils are always used in a diluted form by adding what is called a 'carrier oil' such as almond oil. The essential oils contain plant compounds which are dangerous if swallowed, or even massaged on young children and pregnant women. Also extreme caution should be taken if the patient suffers from any allergic condition such as asthma. Always consult a medically qualified aromatherapist about what oils can be used and what cannot.

Meditation

In the 1950s, Transcendental Meditation was founded by Maharishi Mahesh Yogi in India. After famous celebrities became interested in the subject, it spread worldwide. The main idea behind TM was concentrating on the inner repetition of a personal word or 'mantra' which it was believed could rid the mind of irrelevant thought. Since the 1950s many schools have sprung up having adapted styles and techniques from, in many cases, Eastern philosophies such as Buddha's teaching.

There is scientific evidence that confirms meditation does benefit people. It reduces stress by the metabolic and EEG changes noted during its practise. Research shows a definite heart rate slowing down, the brainwave pattern denotes a mental state combining repose with alertness; at the same time the taking in of oxygen and the depth of breathing decrease and the muscles relax.

It may be that different kinds of meditation may be useful for different purposes or personalities. For instance, 'visualisation' techniques are used in some meditation schools, usually by picturing a shape or colour to let the mind concentrate on. It is used sometimes to fight illness when the patient is taught to 'visualise' the illness and see the body attacking the cancer cells.

'Concentrate meditation' involves gazing or focusing on a static small object, then closing the eyes and trying to visualize the object. Some meditation schools use a lighted candle, it is placed a few feet away at eye level. The gaze should be relaxed, looking steadily but without strain for about one minute before closing the eyes. When the after-image fades, open your eyes and start the process again.

Many recipients have told me that during reflexology treatment they have found themselves doing meditation. It has been my experience to find, if nothing else, meditation can quieten the mind and help us to control, rather then be controlled, by our thoughts and emotions.

Smoking Cessation Therapy

This is not normally listed as a complementary therapy, but in my view, it should be at the top of the list. Whilst working in a hospital as a smoking cessation tutor I concluded that nicotine was one of the greatest health hazards a person would come in contact with. It was also very much apparent that many people who had smoked from adolescence onwards had not learnt to relieve stress in ways that come naturally to non-smokers.

In many cases when I asked a client why they smoked, the answer was, it helped them to relax. In reality this is not so. Nicotine is a mood-altering substance that lasts for a few moments. It raises the blood pressure, increases pulse rate, and the carbon monoxide content of cigarette smoke reduces the levels of oxygen in the blood. Such a state causes the heart to work harder on less oxygen. More than this, it also speeds up furring of the coronary arteries. It becomes a lethal mix, which gradually contributes to heart disease and lung cancer. The ironic fact being that smoking sets the physiological process of stress in motion.

The smoker becomes involved in a complex pattern of behaviour developed over many years, which is habitual. Many of them seem totally unaware of statistics proving that it doubles the risk of dying from a heart attack. In helping clients to quit, I suggested some of the following strategies.

Become highly motivated in wanting to stop. Have a checklist and write down the pros and cons of quitting. See it as quitting one day at a time. Change social situations if you are going to meet in places where smoking will be the norm. Above all, be aware of a greater feeling of better general health, fitness and a sense of well-being.

If giving up becomes a stressful situation then get in touch with one of the health resources in your area that work to helping people give up. Smoking remains the main cause of preventative ill health in Britain, and its related diseases account for thousands of deaths annually.

If you are a smoker reading this book then you are obviously interested in preserving your health. So quit smoking and find yourself; enjoying living more by breathing cleaner air and your food tastes better. If that is not enough, think about how you will lose that hacking cigarette smokers cough. Your sleep will be much sounder and you will feel much less nervous.

If you are a non-smoker, but know of a friend or a family member who smokes then as you practise the therapy with them give encouragement and support to quit. Human empathy and psychological assistance can often mean the difference between success and failure. There will be no doubt they will gain more benefit from R.R. as a non-smoker.

Reference

British Reflexology Association
The Bayly School of Reflexology
Monks Orchard
Whitbourne
Worcester WR6 5RB

Reflexology - A Way To Better Health,
Nicola M Hall
Gateway Books, 1991

The Metamorphic Technique
Gaston Saint-Pierre, and Debbie Shapiro
Element Books 1988

Stories the Feet can Tell
Eunice Ingham Ingham Publishing 1959

International Federation of Aromatherapists
4 Eastmearn Road London SE21 8HA

The Element Family Encyclopaedia of Health
Dr R. Sharma. A complete family reference guide to Alternative and orthodox Medical diagnosis, treatment and preventive Healthcare. Element 1998

The Relaxation Response
Herbert Benson MD and Miriam Z Klipper
Collins 1976

British Homeopathic Association
27a Devonshire Street
London WIN IRJ

British Acupuncture Council
Park House
206-208 Latimer Road
London W10 6RE

The European Shiatsu Network
Highbanks Lockeridge
Marlborough Wiltshire SN8 4TQ

Audio Ltd (biofeedback monitoring devices)
26 Wendall Road
London W12 9rt

Institute for Complementary Medicine
21 Portland Place
London WIN 3AF

Dr Dolores Krieger
The Therapeutic Touch

How to use Your Hands to Help or to Heal
Prentice Hall 1992

QUIT (Action on Smoking and Health)
102 Gloucester Place, London WIH 3DA
Quitline 071 487 3000

James Bevan
Anatomy and Physiology
Mitchell Beazley 1978

Kevin and Barbara Kunz
The Complete Guide to Foot Reflexology
Thorsons 1984

National Carer's Association
29 Chilworth Mews
London W2 3RG

Age Concern
60 Pitcairn Road
Mitcham
Surrey CR4 3LL

Index

A

B

C

D

G

H

I

K

L

M

N

O

P

R

S

T

Z

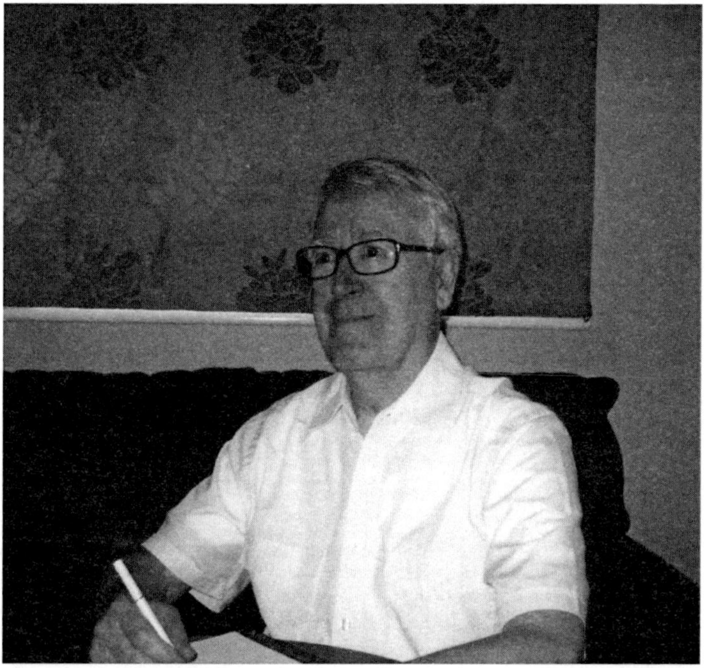

James Brockbank worked in engineering, which included two years in the Armed Forces, and five years for the Ministry of Defence, before training to teach. He did post-graduate study in psychology at Sheffield University and became interested in reflexology whilst working as Headteacher in a special school. He qualified in reflexology at the Bayly School and now lectures extensively in using reflexology for relaxation.

* 9 7 8 1 7 8 0 3 5 0 7 1 4 *

ND - #0185 - 060826 - C0 - 197/132/13 - PB - 9781780350714 - Matt Lamination